SpringerBriefs in Modern Perspectives on Disability Research

Series Editors

Gabriel Bennett, Independent Researcher, Klemzig, Australia

Emma Goodall, Healthy Possibilities, Seaford, Australia

W0037767

This book series on disability research is a comprehensive collection of research on disability and related issues. The series is designed to promote interdisciplinary collaboration and exchange, bringing together scholars and practitioners from different fields to share their perspectives and insights. Disability research is an interdisciplinary field that examines the social, cultural, historical, and political dimensions of disability. It encompasses a wide range of topics, including disability rights, accessibility, assistive technologies, healthcare, education, employment, and social welfare. Disability research scholars employ a range of theoretical and methodological approaches to understand the experiences of people with disabilities, as well as the ways in which disability intersects with other social identities such as race, gender, sexuality, and class.

The series seeks to advance knowledge and understanding of disability by publishing rigorous, innovative, and relevant research. It aims to promote disability rights and social justice by highlighting the ways in which people with disabilities are marginalized and discriminated against in society, and advocating for greater social inclusion and accessibility. The series also seeks to inform policy and practice by disseminating research findings that can help to shape policy decisions and contribute to positive social change.

Vaibhav Sahni

Oral Health in People with Disabilities

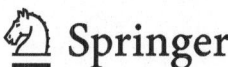 Springer

Vaibhav Sahni
Research and Evidence (RF&E)
New Delhi, Delhi, India

ISSN 3004-9709   ISSN 3004-9717 (electronic)
SpringerBriefs in Modern Perspectives on Disability Research
ISBN 978-981-96-2778-3   ISBN 978-981-96-2779-0 (eBook)
https://doi.org/10.1007/978-981-96-2779-0

This Springer imprint is published by the registered company Springer Nature Singapore Pte Ltd.
The registered company address is: 152 Beach Road, #21-01/04 Gateway East, Singapore 189721,
Singapore

If disposing of this product, please recycle the paper.

To my parents (god) and all those I consider my own kids.

Competing Interests The author has no competing interests to declare that are relevant to the content of this manuscript.

Contents

Abbreviations

AAPD	American Academy of Pediatric Dentistry
ADA	American Dental Association
CP	Cerebral Palsy
DS	Down Syndrome
EHRC	Equality and Human Rights Commission
GIC	Glass Ionomer Cements
HBSS	Hanks' Balanced Salt Solution
MO	Malocclusion
PDL	Periodontal Ligament
SHCN	Special Healthcare Needs
TDI	Traumatic Dental Injury

Introduction

Abstract A significant proportion of the world's population lives with a disability. Each of these individuals faces significant challenges in accessing oral health care. Disabilities present in varying forms and severity making each individual unique in the manner in which they need to be taken care of. There is evidence to suggest that people with disabilities tend to exhibit a greater treatment need for oral health conditions as compared to the general population. This treatment need is expressed for oral diseases and conditions such as caries, periodontal disease, dental trauma and malocclusion. It is imperative for practitioners to understand that each individual's situation is unique in terms of the type, number and severity of disability along with their economic and psychological condition. The dental team and care-givers should take into account accessibility and communication issues along with adapting regular treatment paradigms to suit the unique presentation of these people with special healthcare needs.

Keywords Oral health · Dental · Disability · Special needs

Overview

It has been reported that over a billion people live with a disability of some manner the world over (Leal Rocha et al., 2015). These disabilities vary in their form and severity and in turn affect the general presentation of a patient's condition. Providing care for such individuals is a multi-dimensional issue involving their social and economic considerations, their psychological condition, issues of accessibility (both physical and social), challenges in communication, variety in the presentation of disease processes, underlying medical conditions and comorbidities, adaptation of treatment procedures to their specific needs and ensuring adequate follow-up and commitment of care from the patient and their care-givers.

This book attempts to address these issues by providing the reader with an overview of accessibility and communication strategies in dealing with patients with special healthcare needs. It further goes on to addressing some of the most commonly reported diseases and conditions pertaining to oral health such as dental caries, peri-odontal disease, dental trauma and malocclusion. Each of these topics is dealt with separately in exclusive chapters in a manner which attempts to address the topic solely from the perspective of managing patients with disabilities.

As should be the case in managing such patients, the text does not follow a cookbook approach of providing a certain set of strategies which may be applied to any disease or condition for a patient with any kind of disability. It delves into specific areas of concern and strategies for specific conditions. Naturally, there is bound to be an overlap between certain approaches not only amongst people with disabilities but also between them and the general population. What follows is an overview of the chapters which constitute this book.

Accessibility and Communication

The chapter deals with access-to-care issues encountered by patients while seeking dental care. It deals with the issue of accessibility at different levels such as those encountered in building access, clinic access, dental chair access and access to the mouth itself. These levels are addressed not only in terms of physical challenges but also social and behavioural strategies which can aid in making dental care inclusive and accessible for those with disabilities. The communication section of the chapter provides the reader with an overview of strategies which can be utilised to establish effective communication with people having visual and hearing impairment, aphasia and deafblindness. A number of disabilities present with a varying combination of issues which are attributable to these conditions. In providing strategies of commu-nication for such conditions, it is hoped that the reader will be able to utilise the knowledge to suit the needs of their patients or those under their care.

Periodontal Disease and Disability

Periodontal disease forms a significant burden on the general population which trans-lates into the same for people with disabilities. The issue of periodontal disease is compounded by challenges encountered by those with special healthcare needs in accessing care. Further, periodontal management requires a long-term commitment on part of the patient and their care-givers to maintain home care and follow-up which may be problematic for certain individuals. There is evidence in literature to support the association between periodontal disease and various systemic conditions which further underscores the importance of managing this disease process effec-tively. Treatment strategies and home care regimens need to be individualised to the patient's unique condition along with taking the parents/care-givers into confidence to ensure long-term success.

Dental Caries and Disability

There is conflicting evidence in literature to substantiate whether people with disabilities tend to demonstrate a greater prevalence of dental caries in comparison to the general population. However, evidence also suggests that people with disabilities have a greater number of active and untreated carious lesions which makes the treatment need quite high for this set of the population. Individualised risk assessment strategies help in understanding the unique conditions of the patient and aid in tailoring treatment plans best suited to them. Preference should be granted to preventive/non-restorative treatment modalities over restorative treatment wherever this may be feasible. The eventual aim should be to adapt the treatment to the disabilities of the patient, ensure a positive dental experience and preserve as much of natural dentition as feasible.

Dental Trauma and Disability

In comparison to the general population, there is less literature reporting dental trauma in people with disabilities. It is generally acknowledged that certain conditions may predispose individuals to a higher prevalence of dental trauma as is the case in those with impaired neuromuscular coordination. Another compounding factor to the issues plaguing this topic of research is the fact that management strategies change depending upon whether the traumatised tooth is primary or secondary. Further, literature may tend to report dental trauma in only a particular age group or for a particular disability. This makes the process of arriving at firm conclusions quite tedious. Regardless, the core management strategies for traumatic dental injuries remain the same and these need to be followed with certain adaptations if required, for those presenting with disabilities. The aim should be to not deprive someone of the standard of care simply because they have a disability.

Malocclusion and Disability

Malocclusion or, simply put, problems in the way teeth meet, affect people with disability as well. In fact, certain developmental conditions may predispose these individuals to particular types of malocclusions. Living with a malocclusion can have significant effects on a person's oral function and stability, not to mention their quality of life and visual appearance. These in turn influence an individual's social acceptability and integration. Despite such significant effects on one's overall quality of life and function, orthodontic treatment remains elective. This is attributable to the potential management issues which may arise when dealing with such individuals. Orthodontic treatment takes a protracted course and requires a commitment from the patient as well as the parents/care-givers to ensure compliance and follow-up. Further, it requires a high level of expertise on part of the practitioner to be able to adapt certain components of the treatment plan to suit the individual needs of the patient.

It is hoped that the information in the following chapters will help readers develop a better understanding of managing the oral health of those in their care and, most of all, help arrive at the realisation that those with special needs have to be a tangible part of our society and deserve the same if not a higher standard of health care.

Reference

Leal Rocha, L., Vieira de Lima Saintrain, M., & Pimentel Gomes Fernandes Vieira-Meyer, A. (2015). Access to dental public services by disabled persons. *BMC Oral Health*, 15, 1–9.

Accessibility and Communication

Abstract People living with disabilities encounter a number of accessibility issues be they physical or social. The practitioner, care-givers and society in general need to acknowledge these challenges faced by such individuals and make necessary and reasonable arrangements to aid those living with disabilities in accessing care. These measures can range from physical changes to behavioural ones. In order to ensure cooperation, compliance and any progress in care, an effective communication strategy needs to be employed. People with special needs may present significant challenges as a result of their disabilities and underlying conditions. The practitioner and dental team need to ensure that they are aware of the various strategies they can employ to establish communication with such individuals so as to ensure long-term outcomes of treatment.

Keywords Accessibility · Communication · Oral health · Dental · Deafblind · Aphasia

Introduction

The British Society for Disability and Oral Health (BSDH) has put forth certain guidelines regarding oral health care and developing pathways of integrated oral health care in order to promote equitable care, access and outcomes (Dougall & Fiske, 2008a). A 'case-mix model' tool has been developed with the endorsement of the British Dental Association (BDA) which provides an objective assessment to be conducted for the provision of care complexities for people with disabilities (Dougall & Fiske, 2008a). It aims to assess patient-level complexity instead of dentistry-level complexity by utilising independent criteria which can prove to be determinants either alone or in combination (Dougall & Fiske, 2008a). The criteria considered include communication ability, cooperativeness, medical status, access and oral risk factors along with ethical and legal barriers (Dougall & Fiske, 2008a).

© The Author(s), under exclusive license to Springer Nature Singapore Pte Ltd. 2025
V. Sahni, *Oral Health in People with Disabilities*,
SpringerBriefs in Modern Perspectives on Disability Research,
https://doi.org/10.1007/978-981-96-2779-0_2

The recognition of special care dentistry (SCD) as a standalone speciality is a step in the right direction since it allows for the development and institution of structured training pathways and a workforce to provide care for people with disabilities. Physical access to dental clinics for people with disabilities involves accessibility concerns relating to the building, the clinic itself, the dental chair and the mouth (Dougall & Fiske, 2008a).

Building Access

Physical access to clinics continues to be a significant barrier to care for people with disabilities seeking dental treatment (Baird et al., 2007). The Equality and Human Right Commission (EHRC) recommends that in cases where a person encounters difficulty in accessing a service, the service provider is given the option to alter, remove, find a way to avoid the feature or look into providing a particular service in a different manner (Dougall & Fiske, 2008a). It must be ensured that any alternative should not be unfair or difficult for the person seeking to access the service. In a number of cases ramps and rails will enable access for the majority of individuals with disabilities, and significant building alteration should be made in cases which are deemed reasonable (Dougall & Fiske, 2008a). If a dental practice is not accessible then duty of care dictates that the dentist should arrange reasonable and acceptable alternatives (Dougall & Fiske, 2008a).

In the UK, building regulation and the Disability Discrimination Act (1995) regulate practice design and aim to ensure accessibility for all (Dougall & Fiske, 2008a). Physical aspects are not the only accessibility barriers to dental clinics and attitudes of the staff can have a significant impact. It has been reported that people with disabilities who find the attitudes of the staff amenable tend to be happy with the care they receive as well and that staff attitudes may even go so far as to compensate for certain physical barriers (Dougall & Fiske, 2008a).

Clinic Access

Access audits can help practitioners identify physical barriers that might exist in their practice and help them in making reasonable adjustments to facilitate people with special needs. As a first step, the audit may include seeking the staff and patients' opinion regarding barriers to accessibility for people with disabilities (Dougall & Fiske, 2008a). This can be followed by an appraisal to ascertain which measures are in place and their scope of development or improvement (Dougall & Fiske, 2008a). Certain aspects such as parking, ramps, kerbs, signage and lighting can be looked into along with examining the entrance for a level threshold, width of the doorway, design and position of door handles (Dougall & Fiske, 2008a). The waiting room and reception can be appraised for signage, reception height, seating with wheelchair space and arm rests along with other factors such as the availability of aids for communication and non-slipping floors (Dougall & Fiske, 2008a). The surgery and corridors should avoid any kind of clutter and should provide considerations for wheelchair access. The restrooms should have adequate space, alarms, raised seats and transfer bars (Dougall & Fiske, 2008a).

Dental Chair Access

A consideration should be made to analyse whether the dental chair can provide access for patients of all types or if a 'break-leg' model may be available to facilitate the same (Dougall & Fiske, 2008a). If adequate spacing has been provided in the clinic, the patient can be treated in their own wheelchair or it may be easy for a wheelchair to dental chair transfer to be facilitated (Dougall & Fiske, 2008a; Wilkins, 2004; McGhay, 1980). The former is not ideal in certain cases as it predisposes towards a compromise in posture for both the patient and practitioner (Sasaki et al., 1997; Tamazawa et al., 2004).

It might be helpful to enquire from patients with wheelchairs if they need help with transferring to a dental chair at all since most are able to accomplish this on their own and do not even use a wheelchair all the time (only 5%) (Dougall & Fiske, 2008a). Banana or transfer boards can be used to aid in patient transfer. The board can be placed between the dental chair and wheelchair, and the patient can slide from one to the other (usually by themselves) as a result of the smooth surface of the board (hence, called 'banana') (Dougall & Fiske, 2008a). The staff at the clinic should avoid a manual transfer of the patient from their wheelchair in order to avoid injuries to both themselves and the patient. Ceiling-mounted or foldable hoists can be utilised or even a portable turntable, which is amenable for usage with the majority of dental and wheelchairs particularly in patients with paraplegia (Dougall & Fiske, 2008a; Watt-Smith, 2007).

A dental unit developed in 2004 by a Japanese team allows for mounting a wheelchair or a dental chair (Dougall & Fiske, 2008a). Once the attachment is complete, the chair can be raised, tilted or lowered without compromising posture. Such a design tends to negate any potential accidents which might occur during patient transfer and occupies a similar space in the clinic as conventional units (Dougall & Fiske, 2008a). Another innovative approach is to utilise portable or fixed reclining platforms for wheelchairs which enable the patient to stay in the wheelchair during the visit but are expensive and more suited to high-volume practices (Dougall & Fiske, 2008a).

Oral Access

Access to the mouth may pose a challenge in persons with disabilities, particularly in those lacking the capacity to understand and comprehend their role in the dental treatment. In others, general muscle tone or control or that of the oral apparatus may not be amenable to treatment (Dougall & Fiske, 2008a). In patients with frailty, hypotonia or spasticity, suitable body postures may be created with the use of cushions (Dougall & Fiske, 2008a).

It has been suggested that patients who have spasticity should be positioned in a manner wherein their chin is in close proximity to the chest with the legs and hips separated and in flexion in order to be relaxed (Dougall & Fiske, 2008a). In cases where the specific condition of the patient precludes them from being positioned in such a manner, for example, in Cerebral Palsy (CP) and multiple sclerosis, beanbags and cushions can be utilised (Dougall & Fiske, 2008a). Four cushions developed by the Mun-H-Center in Sweden are designed to be used in the dental chair for the provision of 'non-steady anatomical support' (Dougall & Fiske, 2008a). The cushion with a crescent shape is meant to provide support to the neck, while a ring-shaped 'safe-guarder' can be placed under the neck of the patient and around their arms, back and shoulders (Dougall & Fiske, 2008a). The 'leg-relaxer' can be positioned beneath the knee hollows with its portion to separate the legs being positioned between the knees in order to obviate the leg extension reflex which is particularly helpful in people with spasticity (Dougall & Fiske, 2008a). The feet and calves are supported by the lower leg cushion which also prevents pushing with the feet (Dougall & Fiske, 2008a). The cushions can be used individually or in combination by coupling them with straps of Velcro (Dougall & Fiske, 2008a). The outer surface is washable cotton and the body itself is cleansable with regular or alcohol-based cleaners (Dougall & Fiske, 2008a). Alternatively, travel pillows have also been demonstrated to be effective in providing support in the dental chair (Fiske et al., 2007).

Patients with congestive conditions of the heart and chronic pulmonary illness might require a semi-upright position for the duration of the procedure and a gauge of the degree of reclination required can be made by enquiring the number of cushions the patient needs to sleep (Wilkins & Wilkins, 1976). Arrangements need to be made for patients who might be prone to harming the practitioner or themselves as can be the case with patients with intellectual disabilities, ataxic CP and those with uncontrolled movements of the limbs (Dougall & Fiske, 2008a). Some patients may be predisposed to causing bites upon the practitioner or themselves such as those people with uncontrolled forms of muscle spasms (advanced multiple sclerosis or CP) and those with enhanced bite reflexes (Dougall & Fiske, 2008a). A rubber spatula or bite support (stock or custom) may be utilised in patients prone to biting together (Dougall & Fiske, 2008a). Other measures which may be used in such instances include unbreakable mirror heads and Mckesson props, the latter having the additional benefit of relieving fatigue (Harrell, 2003).

Cheek retractors are also a useful aid in patients with elevated muscle tone or changes in motor functions. They keep the lips and cheek away from the teeth and help keeping the patient's mouth open (Dougall & Fiske, 2008a). They can be used at home to help with toothbrushing and in this manner, familiarise the patient with their presence as well. Certain patients may present with an exaggerated or impaired gag reflex. An impaired gag reflex may be attributed to neurological causes or dysphagia and such patients may have to be positioned upright or semi-upright to avoid aspiration (Fiske et al., 2007). On the other hand, an exaggerated gag reflex can compromise the simplest of intra-oral procedures and the causes have been labelled either psychogenic or somatogenic but usually a combination of these (Dougall & Fiske, 2008a). Certain strategies such as relaxation, distraction, desensitisation and hypnosis along with conscious sedation, Transcutaneous Electrical Nerve Stimulation, acupressure, acupuncture and lastly general anaesthesia (in case all other measures fail) have been suggested to manage an exaggerated gag reflex (Dougall & Fiske, 2008a).

Communication

As is the case with normal patients, effective communication is of great significance in dealing with patients with special needs. This extends further to the parents/guardian/care-givers of such patients as well. Communication with such patients may be hindered by the nature of their disabilities and condition, hence, it is important for people involved in the care of such individuals to recognise these barriers and strategies which can be utilised to communicate effectively.

Visual Impairment

A disability of vision which is not amenable to correction with spectacles is referred to as visual impairment (Dougall & Fiske, 2008b). Individuals with visual impairments can be recognised from carrying a white stick, donning special glasses or having a guide dog accompanying them (Dougall & Fiske, 2008b).

Certain strategies based on tactile feedback can be employed to aid communication with individuals who are visually impaired. These include handshakes, asking the patient to hold one's elbow as they are guided through the clinic, alerting them to the approach of any stairs and informing them of their number (Dougall & Fiske, 2008b).

Any accompanying guide dogs should be allowed inside the clinic. They are trained to not be startled by sudden or loud sounds such as those of aspirators and dental turbines (Dougall & Fiske, 2008b). It should be ensured that any conversation with the patient is done while facing them with no strong lighting at the back as this may cause interferences in their residual vision (Dougall & Fiske, 2008b). The patient should have the procedure described to them and be informed of the steps as they occur, particularly if there is to be a sudden sensation or noise (Dougall & Fiske, 2008b).

To enhance communication with individuals who have a visual impairment, measures such as considering different forms of conveying information should be undertaken such as Braille, spoken word and CDs. The Royal National Institute of Blind People recommends reading standards of large (16–18 font size) or giant print size (anything larger than a large print) (Royal National Institute of Blind People, 2024).

Hearing Impairment

The Royal National Institute for Deaf People recommends certain strategies to help communicate with those who have hearing loss or are deaf. For a start, the person's attention can be drawn towards oneself with a gesture such as waving. It might also be helpful to face the person as a number of them might be dependent on lipreading to aid in understanding. Patience is advocated in such situations and one must be prepared to try new communication strategies or be willing to rephrase or repeat what they are trying to convey. It is also recommended to enquire from someone as to how they wish the communication should be made and this might include involving an interpreter. One can also use device screens with text, paper or whiteboards and pen to write down what one wants to convey. Reducing noise in the background or shifting to quiet surroundings can aid in the communication.

Deaf and Blind

Deafblind UK provides strategies to communicate with people who are both deaf and blind. Such individuals may communicate in a variety of ways which is dependent upon one's own preference and also upon whether a person was born with sensory loss or when they acquired it. Most communication in such cases in non-verbal which relies on voice tone, body language, manual gestures and facial expressions. A number of individuals who are deafblind are able to hear speech if it is clear and talk.

Portable listening devices and hearing aids can obviate the need for lipreading. If a person who is deafblind relies on lipreading for aiding in communication, one should make sure they are positioned in a manner that they can be seen while communicating and their hands are not around or over their mouth. Patients who are deafblind might prefer to communicate in sign language (British sign language, signed English, Makaton/key word signing, visual frame signing) which uses manual gestures. People who have further low vision may utilise a tactile version of sign language which necessitates feeling the signer's hand movements. The Deafblind Manual by Deafblind

UK involves signing letters individually onto one's hands so one is able to spell these. 'Block' involves drawing capital letters in English onto one's palm. Another method of tactile communication is Braille which utilises a series of elevated dots which can be felt. It was originally used with embossed paper but can now be used with Braille displays which are refreshable. Tadoma may be utilised by certain individuals which involves placing one's hand on someone's lips, cheeks or throat to feel movements of the lip and vibrations. Another tactile system of writing but one seldom used these days is 'Moon' which follows visually recognisable letter formation in English in place of Braille-like dots. Some patients may utilise objects of reference as a method of communication, and this might be helpful in establishing particular objects to signal different phases of the dental appointment.

Aphasia

Aphasia refers to an impairment in communication which is acquired as a result of damage to the parts of the brain which are responsible for producing speech. The National Aphasia Association provides certain suggestions to help in communication with people with Aphasia. It is recommended that one ensures they have the attention of the individual before any communication is started. Any background noise should be eliminated or minimised. When communicating with a person with aphasia, one should avoid being condescending but keep their communication adult and simple with a reduced speech rate. One's voice level should remain at its normal levels unless the person with aphasia indicates otherwise. Individuals with aphasia should be provided the time and opportunity to speak, and one must not rush to offer suggestions or finish their sentences. One can check if the communication is successful by asking simple questions with a 'yes' or 'no' answer. Gestures, drawing, facial expressions and writing can be used in addition to spoken word. One should avoid being critical of the speech an individual with aphasia is able to produce and avoid being overprotective of them, and encourage their integration into normal activities and their independence.

References

Baird, W. O., McGrother, C., Abrams, K. R., Dugmore, C., & Jackson, R. J. (2007). Verifiable CPD paper: Factors that influence the dental attendance pattern and maintenance of oral health for people with multiple sclerosis. *British Dental Journal, 202*(1), E4–41. https://doi.org/10.1038/bdj.2006.125.

Dougall, A., & Fiske, J. (2008a). Access to special care dentistry, part 1. Access. *British Dental Journal, 204*(11), 605–616. https://doi.org/10.1038/sj.bdj.2008.457.

Dougall, A., & Fiske, J. (2008b). Access to special care dentistry, part 2. Communication. *British Dental Journal, 205*(1), 11–21. https://doi.org/10.1038/sj.bdj.2008.533.

Fiske, J., Dickinson, C., Boyle, C., Rafique, S., & Boyle, M. (2007). Managing the health of patients with physical disabilities. *Special Care Dentistry*, 9–26.

Harrell, S. N. (2003). Managing slightly uncooperative pediatric patients. *The Journal of the American Dental Association, 134*(12), 1613–1614.

McGhay, R. M. (1980). A simple headrest for patients confined to wheelchairs. *The Journal of Prosthetic Dentistry, 44*(3), 347–349. https://doi.org/10.1016/0022-3913(80)90026-8.

Royal National Institute of Blind People. (2024). https://www.rnib.org.uk/living-with-sight-loss/independent-living/reading-and-books/large-and-giant-print/.

Sasaki, K., Watanabe, M., & Tamazawa, Y. (1997). A special clinic for the elderly at a centre of dental clinics. *Gerodontology, 11*, 281–282.

Tamazawa, Y., Watanabe, M., Kikuchi, M., Takatsu, M., Tamazawa, K., Yumoto, N., & Hyvarinen, P. (2004). A new dental unit for both patients in wheelchairs and general patients. *Gerodontology, 21*(1), 53–59. https://doi.org/10.1111/j.1741-2358.2004.00011.x.

Watt-Smith, P., & Walton, G. (2007). A case study on the use of turntable transfer. *J Disabil Oral Health, 8*, 132–134.

Wilkins, E. M. (2004). Patients with special needs. In: *Clinical practice of the dental hygienist* (9th ed). Section 7. Philadelphia: Lippincott, Williams & Wilkins.

Wilkins, E. M., & Wilkins. (1976). *Clinical practice of the dental hygienist* (pp. 273–283). Philadelphia: Lea & Febiger.

Periodontal Disease and Disability

Abstract Periodontal disease affects a considerable proportion of not only the general population but also those living with disabilities. There is evidence in literature to suggest the association of periodontal disease with systemic conditions which further emphasises the importance of management. People with special needs face accessibility issues in terms of oral health care, and this might further create problems in treating periodontal disease seeing as it requires a long-term commitment from both the practitioner's and patient's end. Treatment strategies and home care need to be tailored to the patient's specific needs while taking the parent or care-giver into confidence so as to ensure successful long-term outcomes.

Keywords Periodontal disease · Disability · Oral hygiene · Periodontitis · Gingivitis

Periodontal Disease

Periodontal disease includes, within its ambit, numerous chronic inflammatory disease processes pertaining to the gums (gingiva), periodontal ligament (connective tissue which connects the teeth to the alveolar bone) and alveolar bone (the part of the jaw bone housing the tooth) (Kinane et al., 2017). Periodontal disease etiology is considered to be multifactorial in nature, which is both polymicrobial and host-specific (Sahni & Van Dyke, 2023). An initial microbial insult may initiate the disease process; however, it is the inflammatory response of the host which is responsible for further pathogenesis (Sahni & Van Dyke, 2023). Periodontitis is considered to be an inflammatory disease which possesses a bacterial initiation, according to the American Academy of Periodontology (Sahni & Van Dyke, 2023). It is still unclear, though, whether said inflammatory response occurs prior to the dysbiosis or the other way around (Sahni & Van Dyke, 2023).

Generally, the periodontal disease process is initiated with a localised gingival inflammation caused by bacteria residing in consonance with dental plaque. This condition is termed *gingivitis* (Kinane et al., 2017). If gingivitis remains untreated, it may lead to a loss of periodontal ligament, bone and gingiva (Periodontitis) which in turn forms 'periodontal pockets', eventually leading to tooth loss (Kinane et al., 2017). The effects of this inflammatory burden may also be manifested at a systemic level to involve other disease processes such as atherosclerosis and diabetes mellitus (Kinane et al., 2017).

Chronic periodontitis can be classified as generalised or localised based on the number of teeth involved. Where greater than ten teeth of the thirty-two in a dentition are involved the condition is termed generalised, and a count below ten is termed localised (Kinane et al., 2017). Periodontal diseases also involve other conditions such as peri-implant mucositis and peri-implantitis which pertain to the connective tissue surrounding dental implants and involve the peri-implant mucosa and peri-implant bone loss respectively. Destruction of periodontal tissue may also manifest in consonance with syndromic conditions such as Papillon-Lefèvre syndrome, Chediak-Higashi syndrome and leukocyte adhesion deficiency (Kinane et al., 2017). Necrotising forms of the disease also occur, which are necrotising ulcerative gingivitis and necrotising ulcerative periodontitis which tend to occur in debilitated patients and involve a rapid progression of tissue destruction (Kinane et al., 2017).

The new 2017 classification system of periodontal diseases introduces significant changes to the previous 1999 system. The 'aggressive' form of periodontitis has now been omitted as it was acknowledged that there is no evidence in literature to distinguish this form of disease from the chronic variant. The new system has also introduced the concept of staging (disease severity and management complexity) and grading (denotes supplemental details pertaining to biological features), maintains the category of necrotising disease forms, defines gingival recession in terms of clinical attachment loss in the inter-proximal region, excludes the term periodontal biotype in favour of periodontal phenotype and replaces the term excessive occlusal force with traumatic occlusal force to emphasise forces exceeding the adaptive limits of the teeth or periodontium; the term biologic width is replaced by supracrestal attachment, and peri-implant conditions and diseases are categorised separately under the categories of peri-implant health, peri-implantitis and peri-implant mucositis.

Clinical Assessment of Periodontal Features

The assessment of the periodontium involves a number of clinical features which are generally assessed visually with some being supplemented with measurements. The gingival colour and contour are assessed upon inspection by the examiner, the gingival phenotype (erstwhile biotype) gauges tissue transparency upon probing, and recession and pocket depth measurements are made using periodontal probes which can then be used to evaluate attachment loss. Bleeding on probing is a hallmark of inflammation and ascertained upon visual inspection. Mobility of the dentition can be evaluated visually along with using indices such as Miller's index to categorise these into varying levels of severity. Furcation involvement of the dentition may be assessed with a probe and supplemented with indices. Other features such as those pertaining to the presence and location of plaque, calculus and pus may be evaluated upon visual inspection and supplemented with indices as deemed relevant.

The Status of Periodontal Disease in People with Special Needs

The 2000 US Surgeon General's report informed that patients with special healthcare needs are disproportionately affected by periodontal disease in comparison to the rest of the population. Patients with dementia, post-traumatic stress, depression, learning difficulties, poor mobility and psychiatric disorders may be at an elevated risk of being susceptible to periodontal disease.

A study involving 832 participants from 10 schools found worse levels of oral hygiene and an increased prevalence of periodontal disease in people with disabilities (DS, hearing-disabled, visually disabled, physically disabled) when compared to children without disability. Another study which included 4732 adults with developmental and learning disabilities found periodontitis in 80.3% of the cohort with the prevalence being highest (92.6%) in those over the age of 60 years, while the lowest prevalence (55.8%) was observed in the age group of 20–39 years. The authors flagged cooperability, age and residence status as being significant factors in charting preventive management strategies in this cohort which demonstrated a high burden of disease (Morgan et al., 2012).

A systematic review found a strong association between Down Syndrome (DS) and periodontitis, whereas that between DS and gingivitis was found to be moderate. Generally, it has been acknowledged that people with DS are more susceptible to periodontal disease both in terms of prevalence and severity. In a study assessing the periodontal status of 70 children (10.8 ± 3 years) with DS, it was found that periodontal disease was present in 96% of the cohort and presented with greater severity in this group when compared to non-DS age-matched controls with learning disabilities (Johnson & Young, 1963). A number of studies have demonstrated a horizontal pattern of bone loss in the mandibular anterior region in DS patients (Agholme et al., 1999; Cichon et al., 1998; Johnson & Young, 1963; Saxén et al., 1977). A number of people with DS tend to be under institutional care. It has been reported that institutionalised people with DS have worse plaque control levels, greater calculus deposits and increased periodontal disease prevalence in comparison to people with DS who live at home (Morgan, 2007).

A number of etiological factors have been identified for periodontal disease occurring in DS patients. These may be grouped in local and systemic factors. The local factors include poor oral hygiene (Cohen, 1960; Sakellari et al., 2001; Barr-Agholme et al., 1998), mouth breathing due to maxillary hypoplasia, a prognathic mandible and increased tonsillar volume (Morgan, 2007). Another local factor is tooth morphology wherein smaller and shorter tooth dimensions along with fused roots in multi-rooted teeth have been espoused to contribute to periodontal disease in DS patients (Morgan,

2007). It has also been observed that DS patients tend to exhibit significantly greater levels of periodontopathogens such as *P. intermedia, T. forsythia, A. actinomycetem-comitans* and *P. gingivalis* (Sakellari et al., 2005). *P. gingivalis* in particular has been observed to increase in occurrence as age progresses (Morgan, 2007). Herpes virus species such as human cytomegalovirus, Epstein-Barr virus and herpes simplex virus have also been found to be related to periodontal pathology in DS patients at subgingival sites (Hanookai et al., 2000). DS patients have also been demonstrated to suffer from necrotising forms of periodontal disease. There is evidence in literature to suggest that DS patients may suffer from at least one to multiple episodes of acute nectrotising ulcerative gingivitis and that this disease process may occur at earlier stages in life (9.4 ± 4.4 years) as compared to people without DS in whom it tends to occur in young adulthood (Cohen et al., 1961; Harvey Brown, 1973; Morgan, 2007).

Systemic factors such as neutrophil dysfunction have been demonstrated to play a role in the pathophysiology of periodontal disease in DS patients. Being the natural first line of defence, neutrophils have been observed to accumulate at sites of challenge at varying stages of periodontal disease. Neutrophils have cell surface receptors which help them to attach and phagocytose bacteria. There is evidence of an impairment of neutrophil chemotaxis and phagocytosis in DS patients (Izumi et al., 1989; Yavuzyilmaz et al., 1993). This dysfunction may be attributable to the shorter half-life of neutrophils in DS patients (3.7 h) versus that in the healthy population (6.6 h) (Yavuzyilmaz et al., 1993). T-lymphocyte dysfunction in terms of a dwindled recognition and responsive capacity, increased activity of proteolytic enzymes and inflammatory mediators and inflammation as a function of hyperinnervation have also been implicated in the causality of periodontal disease in this group of patients (Morgan, 2007).

People with DS are prone to the development of extensive gingivitis at early stages of life which may progress to periodontal disease of a rapidly progressing nature by the time they reach young adulthood which is marked by severe forms of mobility in the dentition and eventual tooth loss as early as the end of the fourth decade of life (Brown et al., 2017). Clinically, this elevated susceptibility to periodontal disease is highlighted by more bleeding on probing, greater number of missing teeth and increased gingival and plaque indices, which is along the same lines as individuals with mental disability (Brown et al., 2017). Indeed, cognitive impairment has been found to be associated with edentulism, increased number of carious dentition and poor hygiene of dentures (Syrjälä A-MH 2007).

In keeping with similar trends, conditions involving physical impairments such as Rheumatoid arthritis, multiple sclerosis and Parkinson's disease have been demonstrated to be associated with severe forms of periodontal disease. Individuals with Parkinson's disease have been observed to undergo increased levels of gingival recession, and possess worse oral health, greater bleeding on probing, deeper levels of periodontal pockets, worse oral hygiene and elevated mobility of the dentition (Brown et al., 2017). Recently, periodontal disease and Rheumatoid arthritis have been observed to possess a likely association based on a common pathophysiological pathway (Kaur et al., 2013).

An increased incidence of periodontal disease and mandibular dysfunction has been reported in patients of Rheumatoid arthritis. The accompanying sequelae of the disease, such as pain and deviation of digits, joint swelling and digit stiffness may interfere with proper oral care such as that which involves interdental cleaning and even toothbrushing (Brown et al., 2017).

Individuals living with social disability such as prisoners, the homeless, individuals with a mental illness and people of a low socioeconomic status may also be at a greater risk of suffering from oral disease(s). It has been acknowledged that those at the more severe end of social disability are particularly vulnerable towards poor oral health as well as overall health due to impediments in access to care. There exists a social gradient in terms of both oral and overall health wherein increased social advantage associates with worse health-related outcomes (Sabbah et al., 2007).

According to the NHANES III (the third National Health and Nutrition Examination Survey), periodontal disease had a greater prevalence in individuals educated for less than twelve years (30.7%) as compared to those educated for more than twelve years (18.6%) (Sabbah et al., 2007). This is clear evidence of the existence of a social gradient for an individual's periodontal status.

Homeless individuals face significant challenges in terms of accessing care due to the complexity of medical, social and psychological factors they encounter. Certain factors such as absence of social support, poverty, substance abuse and mental illness need to be considered in the management of such individuals (Brown et al., 2017). Despite the challenges of collecting data in such population groups, studies indicate that homeless individuals demonstrate a high treatment need for periodontal disease (71 and 80% of participants in two separate studies) (Daly et al., 2010; Ford et al., 2014).

Individuals suffering from severe forms of mental illness have been demonstrated to possess poorer oral health-related quality of life and oral health as compared to the population in general. Improper oral hygiene practices, inadequate dietary care, diabetes and smoking can further compound oral health issues. Antipsychotic medications have been known to cause dryness of the mouth which can have severe consequences for the health of the oral cavity. Barriers to access, a downslide in self-care and other medical conditions may lead to an assignment of low priority to oral health in such patients (Brown et al., 2017).

Periodontal Disease and Quality of Life

It has been acknowledged that the effects of periodontal disease on the quality of life has been evaluated in fewer studies when compared to other diseases of the oral cavity (El Tantawi et al., 2017). Periodontal disease can have negative effects on the overall quality of life exerting functional limitations, causing pain as well as psychological and physical discomfort (El Tantawi et al., 2017). People with disabilities may have mental or physical conditions which limit or affect their daily living and as such may warrant special accommodation. Poor oral health can involve loss of dentition, pain, malnutrition, difficulty in speech, malodor, deteriorated appearance and financial constraints (Brown et al., 2017). It may give rise to situations where individuals with disabilities may be isolated thereby impeding their social acceptance and integration.

Difference in the Management of Periodontal Disease for Special Needs Patients

Data from the Census Bureau indicated that by the end of 1994, twenty six million people were living with a severe form of disability while more than double this number (fifty four million) had at least some form of disability (Waldman et al., 2000). The chances of severe disability increase as age advances with children (6–14 years of age) at 1.9%, adults (55–64 years of age) at 36.3% and the elderly (over 80 years of age) at 53.5% (Waldman et al., 2000). It has been reported for the population above six years of age that 5.2 million have to utilise crutches, a cane or a walker and have used these for a period of six months or more (Waldman et al., 2000). A further 1.8 million reportedly utilise a wheelchair with 8.8 million people in this age group having difficulty in vision (which includes the 1.6 million blind individuals) (Waldman et al., 2000). Activities of daily living include amongst them acts such as those of getting out of or into a chair or bed, going around the house, dressing, bathing, toileting and eating (Waldman et al., 2000). Literature suggests that at the end of 1994, there were 4.1 million people who were in need of assistance with such activities (Waldman et al., 2000).

In people aged twenty-two years and above, it has been reported that severe disabilities affect a greater number of females as compared to males, while a greater percentage of Hispanics and black non-Hispanics had severe disabilities as compared to white non-Hispanics (McNeil, 1997). These statistics clearly suggest a vast, expanding set of issues which need consideration in terms of the provision of oral health care to people with disabilities.

The eventual outcome of a periodontal treatment plan is, for the large part, dependent upon the motivation and ability of the individual being rendered the treatment, or, in the case of people with disabilities, that of care-givers and/or parents (Waldman et al., 2000). Certain points need to be borne in mind while devising the treatment plan for individuals with disabilities, such as behaviour management which refers to the ability of the patient to comply with the treatment plan. The ability of the patient to maintain oral hygiene up to a desired level needs to be considered along with the motivation and willingness of the patient towards the treatment being rendered (Waldman et al., 2000). It is imperative for the general public and practitioners alike to recognise the wide variation of disabilities certain individuals may be living with. Instead of utilising the broad label of a 'disability' on a history form and introducing a vague, possibly stereotypical image, practitioners should consider the varying nature of disabilities while formulating treatment plans.

There is a dearth of literature regarding periodontal treatment outcomes in patients with special needs. A study which analysed oral health-related outcomes over a twelve-year time period in an adult population with developmental and learning disabilities found that caries prevalence reduced while that of periodontitis increased (Finkelman et al., 2014).

Access and Provision of Care

Over a quarter of a million people with developmental disabilities or mental retardation were in state institutions as of 1967, which included 34,000 diagnosed people in psychiatric institutions and 195,650 individuals in state institutions for people diagnosed with developmental disabilities or mental retardation (Waldman et al., 2000). The next thirty years saw a decline in the total of institutionalised people by 75% which meant that by 1997, 57,200 people remained in institutional care (Waldman et al., 2000). Further, people institutionalised in psychiatric institutions underwent a decrease of 97% to a total of 1075 people in such institutional care (Waldman et al., 2000).

This de-institutionalisation has led to a more complex situation of oral health-care access (Brown et al., 2017). The severity of disability tends to increase as age advances, and the fact that people with special care needs may have varying living conditions ranging from residing in their own home to being homeless may further compound the problem of access to care. Worsening severity of the disability along with the presence of multiple types of disabilities may render this population especially vulnerable. The compromise in oral health may be the result of one or several factors acting at different levels. It may be due to conditions leading to compromised oral function/structures, due to the medical line of management of the disability which predisposes towards oral health compromise or as a direct result of the disability itself which may leave an individual socially compromised and hinder access to care (Brown et al., 2017).

General dental practitioners (GDPs) may opt to refer such patients to specialists such as a periodontist or those in special care dentistry. This may be the result of a lack of experience and/or training on part of the GDPs (Brown et al., 2017). Other factors posing barriers to access to care for people with disabilities may include lack of an ideally equipped clinical setup, the ability/confidence/willingness of GDPs to deal with such cases, patient disability management during the procedure, lack of appropriate oral access to satisfactorily render treatment, finances and the duration of the dental appointment itself (Bateman et al., 2010; Dougall & Fiske, 2008).

Certain patient-level factors may also tend to compromise periodontal management in people with disabilities. Such patient groups have been noted to demonstrate a greater incidence of malocclusions when compared to the normal population (Waldman et al., 2000). This, in turn, is related to craniofacial anomalies, anomalous development and growth, disturbances in orofacial musculature and anomalous tongue posture (Waldman et al., 2000). Further, these patients may be multiply medicated which can have undesirable side effects compromising oral care. Gingival hyperplasia may arise as a result of seizure medications. Another pertinent condition is that of dry mouth usually caused as a result of cardiovascular and psychotropic medication (Waldman et al., 2000). Patients with mental retardation may be unable to fully comprehend the necessity of oral hygiene maintenance while those with physical disabilities may not have sufficient dexterity to perform oral care (Waldman et al., 2000).

Patients presenting with complex forms of medical conditions may necessitate management in the multidisciplinary team (including dental hygienists, dentists and oral health therapists with referrals to specialists where required) format within a hospital setting under general anaesthesia (Brown et al., 2017).

Such situations may further be complicated by the patient's inability to cooperate and communicate sufficiently to provide consent (Brown et al., 2017). A successful approach towards treating patients with special needs has been to subject standard treatment protocols to slight modifications to suit the varying needs of these groups (Waldman et al., 2000). The guardian/parents may be requested to assume complete responsibility for the maintenance of oral hygiene and preventive measures for caries (Waldman et al., 2000).

By ensuring such steps are in place along with frequent assessments during the course of treatment may lead to successful delivery of treatment to those with special needs. The practitioner's positive attitude has been demonstrated to elevate the chances of treatment provision to underserved people (Brown et al., 2017). For continued maintenance of oral health, it is equally important for the care-giver to be educated and motivated in order to enhance long-term outcomes and regular dental visits.

Individualised Approach to Periodontal Management

It is a well-recognised fact that the nature and severity of disability and its accompanying social and medical factors need to be considered while devising treatment plans for such individuals. As such, this precludes a cookbook approach, with treatment ideally being tailored to suit the specific needs of patients presenting with disabilities.

History

It is important for the practitioner to establish effective and empathetic communication with the care-giver and take into account issues such as the level of literacy being dealt with, consent and laws governing patient privacy. It is also important to record the oral hygiene habits a patient is able to follow and whether any of these require assistance along with the level of assistance needed. The history must also make specific notes of any medications the patient may be on along with their medical and dental history.

Examination

The practitioner and staff should be sanguine with the fact that such patients may require prolonged appointment times and even multiple appointments. The clinical setup must be enabled for accessibility to the dental chair with assistance available should it be required either in terms of manpower or equipment. In case special equipment is installed, it should be compliant with occupational health and safety guidelines.

During the examination procedure, certain factors such as macroglossia as well as the presence or absence of a gag reflex should be borne in mind and care should be taken that the patient does not inadvertently inhale or ingest foreign objects. The quality and quantity of salivary secretions also need to be noted as it may effect further care and rendering of treatment. Plaque retentive features and parafunctional habits must be identified. Care should be taken that the patient is comfortable during positioning for intra-oral radiography and panoramic or three-dimensional alternatives may be considered.

Diagnosis

The diagnosis should take into account any underlying medical conditions, and it must be carefully noted whether the findings of an examination constitute a syndromic presentation. The practitioner should at this stage evaluate the effects of other medical conditions on the delivery of care.

Preventive Periodontal Management

Any programme of preventive care being instituted should be individualised to the patient's specific needs. Visual aids such as photographs and plaque disclosing agents may be utilised for care-giver/patient education. Proper instructions to the care-giver or patient can go a long way in helping them maintain oral hygiene, which can include a variety of methods such as mouthrinses, interdental aids and electric/manual toothbrushes. Smoking and other deleterious habits should also be addressed in this phase of treatment along with providing nutrition counselling.

Non-surgical Periodontal Treatment

The rendering of treatment may be staggered in phases to make it tolerable for the patient. The appointment time should suit both the patient and the practitioner with the possibility of extension if deemed necessary. Dentition with poor prognosis should be removed, and procedures under general anaesthesia may include full mouth debridement.

Review

The patient may be reviewed in three to six months' time wherein an examination of previous charting, and reviewing the medical history, oral hygiene, smoking status and diet may be undertaken. A note must also be made to signify any changes in the status of the patient's arrangements of care.

Maintenance

The patient and/or care-giver's ability to maintain their oral hygiene should influence the period of recall. The dental practitioner should review the case and involve the care-giver/patient to maintain oral hygiene with professional maintenance being performed by hygienists.

Surgical Treatment

Any surgical treatment being considered must be preceded by an open and thorough discussion with the patient and care-giver regarding its perceived benefits and sequelae as well as possible complications. The level of home care required post-surgery must be impressed upon the patient and care-giver in order to empower them and ensure they are involved in the treatment process.

Emergency Treatment

Pain or infection must be addressed in as urgent a manner as possible with consideration being made for antibiotic administration in patients who may be immuno-suppressed. Prompt specialist referral or management in a hospital setting may be necessitated in certain cases and should be implemented without hesitation.

Conclusion

People with disabilities are more prone to periodontal compromise and face significant challenges in terms of access to care, undergoing treatment and maintenance of oral hygiene. The provision of periodontal care to patients with special needs requires empathy and cooperation both on part of the patient/care-giver as well as the practitioner. Such patients should have thorough examinations and prompt referrals where required, taking into account the number and severity of their disabilities. Underlying medical conditions in such patients also affect the type and delivery of care and should be considered throughout the management process.

References

Agholme, M. B., Dahllof, G., & Modéer, T. (1999). Changes of periodontal status in patients with Down syndrome during a 7-year period. *European journal of oral sciences, 107*(2).

Barr-Agholme, M., Dahllöf, G., Modéer, T., Engström, P. E., & Engström, G. N. (1998). Periodontal conditions and salivary immunoglobulins in individuals with Down syndrome. *Journal of Periodontology, 69*(10), 1119–1123.

Bateman, P., Arnold, C., Brown, R., Foster, L. V., Greening, S., Monaghan, N., & Zoitopoulos, L. (2010). BDA special care case mix model. *British Dental Journal, 208*(7), 291–296.

Brown, L. F., Ford, P. J., & Symons, A. L. (2017). Periodontal disease and the special needs patient. *Periodontology 2000, 74*(1), 182–193. https://doi.org/10.1111/prd.12198.

Caton, J. G., Armitage, G., Berglundh, T., Chapple, I. L., Jepsen, S., Kornman, K. S., & Tonetti, M. S. (2018). A new classification scheme for periodontal and peri-implant diseases and conditions–introduction and key changes from the 1999 classification. *Journal of Periodontology, 89*, S1–S8.

Cichon, P., Crawford, L., & Grimm, W. D. (1998). Early-onset periodontitis associated with down's syndrome–a clinical interventional study. *Annals of Periodontology, 3*(1), 370–380.

Cohen, M. (1960). Periodontal disease in a group of mentally subnormal children. *Journal of Dental Research, 39*, 745.

Cohen, M. M., Winer, R. A., Schwartz, S., & Shklar, G. (1961). Oral aspects of mongolism: Part I. Periodontal disease in mongolism. *Oral Surgery, Oral Medicine, Oral Pathology, 14*(1), 92–107.

Daly, B., Newton, T., Batchelor, P., & Jones, K. (2010). Oral health care needs and oral health-related quality of life (OHIP-14) in homeless people. *Community Dentistry and Oral Epidemiology, 38*(2), 136–144.

Dougall, A., & Fiske, J. (2008). Access to special care dentistry, part 9. Special care dentistry services for older people. *British dental journal, 205*(8), 421–434.

El Tantawi, M., & AlAgl, A. (2017). Disability and the impact of need for periodontal care on quality of life: A cross-sectional study. *Journal of International Medical Research, 45*(6), 1949–1960. https://doi.org/10.1177/0300060517715376

Finkelman, M. D., Stark, P. C., Tao, W., & Morgan, J. P. (2014). Relationship between duration of treatment and oral health in adults with intellectual and developmental disabilities. *Special Care in Dentistry, 34*(4).

Ford, P. J., Cramb, S., & Farah, C. S. (2014). Oral health impacts and quality of life in an urban homeless population. *Australian Dental Journal, 59*(2), 234–239.

Hanookai, D., Nowzari, H., Contreras, A., Morrison, J. L., & Slots, J. (2000). Herpesviruses and periodontopathic bacteria in Trisomy 21 periodontitis. *Journal of Periodontology, 71*(3), 376–384.

Harvey Brown, R. (1973). Necrotizing ulcerative gingivitis in mongoloid and non-mongoloid retarded individuals. *Journal of Periodontal Research, 8*(5), 290–295.

Izumi, Y., Sugiyama, S., Shinozuka, O., Yamazaki, T., Ohyama, T., & Ishikawa, I. (1989). Defective neutrophil chemotaxis in Down's syndrome patients and its relationship to periodontal destruction. *Journal of periodontology, 60*(5), 238–242. https://doi.org/10.1902/jop.1989.60.5.238.

Johnson, N. P., & Young, M. A. (1963). Periodontal disease in mongols. *The Journal of Periodontology, 34*(1), 41–47.

Kaur, S., White, S., & Bartold, P. M. (2013). Periodontal disease and rheumatoid arthritis: A systematic review. *Journal of Dental Research, 92*(5), 399–408.

Kinane, D. F., Stathopoulou, P. G., & Papapanou, P. N. (2017). Periodontal diseases. *Nature Reviews Disease Primers, 3*(1), 1–14.

McNeil, J. (1997). Americans with Disabilities: 1994–95. Washington, DC; United States Bureau of the Census. Retrieved April 12, 2001 from http://www.blue.census.gov/hhes/www/disable/sipp/disab9495/oldasc.htm.

Milward, M. R., & Roberts, A. (2019). Assessing periodontal health and the British society of periodontology implementation of the new classification of periodontal diseases 2017. *Dental Update, 46*(10), 918–929.

Morgan, J. (2007). Why is periodontal disease more prevalent and more severe in people with Down syndrome? *Special Care in Dentistry, 27*(5), 196–201.

Morgan, J. P., Minihan, P. M., Stark, P. C., Finkelman, M. D., Yantsides, K. E., Park, A., Nobles, C. J., Tao, W., & Must, A. (2012). The oral health status of 4,732 adults with intellectual and developmental disabilities. *Journal of the American Dental Association (1939), 143*(8), 838–846. https://doi.org/10.14219/jada.archive.2012.0288.

Rondón-Avalo, S., Rodríguez-Medina, C., & Botero, J. E. (2024). Association of Down syndrome with periodontal diseases: Systematic review and meta-analysis. *Special Care in Dentistry: Official Publication of the American Association of Hospital Dentists, the Academy of Dentistry for the Handicapped, and the American Society for Geriatric Dentistry, 44*(2), 360–368. https://doi.org/10.1111/scd.12892.

Sabbah, W., Tsakos, G., Chandola, T., Sheiham, A., & Watt, R. G. (2007). Social gradients in oral and general health. *Journal of Dental Research, 86*(10), 992–996.

Sahni, V., & Van Dyke, T. E. (2023). Immunomodulation of periodontitis with SPMs. *Frontiers in Oral Health, 4*, 1288722. https://doi.org/10.3389/froh.2023.1288722.

Sakellari, D., Arapostathis, K. N., & Konstantinidis, A. (2005). Periodontal conditions and subgingival microflora in Down syndrome patients: A case—control study. *Journal of Clinical Periodontology, 32*(6), 684–690.

Sakellari, D., Belibasakis, G., Chadjipadelis, T., Arapostathis, K., & Konstantinidis, A. (2001). Supragingival and subgingival microbiota of adult patients with Down's syndrome. Changes after periodontal treatment. *Oral Microbiology and Immunology, 16*(6), 376–382.

Saxén, L., Aula, S., & Westermarck, T. (1977). Periodontal disease associated with Down's syndrome: An orthopantomographic evaluation. *Journal of Periodontology, 48*(6), 337–340.

Shyama, M., Al-Mutawa, S. A., Honkala, S., Sugathan, T., & Honkala, E. (2000). Oral hygiene and periodontal conditions in special needs children and young adults in Kuwait. *J Disabil Oral Health, 1*, 13–19.

Syrjälä A-MH. (2007). Relationship between cognitive impairment and oral health: Results of the Health 2000 Health Examination Survey in Finland. *Acta Odontol, 65*, 103–108.

Yavuzyilmaz, E., Ersoy, F., Sanal, O., Tezcan, I., & Erçal, D. (1993). Neutrophil chemotaxis and periodontal status in Down's syndrome patients. *The Journal of Nihon University School of Dentistry, 35*(2), 91–95. https://doi.org/10.2334/josnusd1959.35.91.

Dental Caries and Disability

Abstract Dental caries represents a significant unmet treatment need in people living with disabilities. Each individual with special needs presents with a unique condition in terms of the type and severity of their disability as well as their socioeconomic and psychological situation. This mandates the utilisation of individualised risk assessment strategies. The treatment for carious lesions should prefer preventive strategies and non-restorative measures over restorative treatment paradigms with the ultimate goal being to preserve as much of natural dentition as is reasonably possible.

Keywords Dental caries · Restorative treatment · Prevention · Non-restorative treatment

Introduction

Dental caries is a non-communicable disease with a multifactorial aetiology and remains a significant public health concern across various population and age groups despite advances in its management (Campos & Fontana, 2022). Though there is conflicting data to contest this, it is generally acknowledged that people with special healthcare needs (SHCNs) are at a greater risk of developing caries. In the case of children, however, a recent systematic review and meta-analysis concluded that there appeared to be no evidence to suggest a different level of caries in the primary or permanent dentition of children living with learning disabilities as compared to those without (Robertson et al., 2019). There was, though, evidence of lower caries levels in Down's syndrome (DS) children, but the same was not evident in those with mixed learning disabilities or autism (Robertson et al., 2019).

Overall, people with disabilities have been reported to demonstrate a greater prevalence of untreated and active carious lesions, challenges to maintain oral hygiene and difficulty in access to care which may lead to unaddressed dental needs (Robertson et al., 2019; de Azeredo et al., 2019; Khalid et al., 2019; Pini et al., 2016). The situation is further compounded by the unique condition of each person with a disability which involves factors relating to socioeconomics, motor skills, demographics, psychological and behavioural (Campos & Fontana, 2022).

Risk Assessment

Risk assessment for caries is of importance in prevention as well as the subsequent therapeutic management, informing treatment strategies and estimating prognosis (Campos & Fontana, 2022). Periodic assessments of caries risk may be a helpful strategy in devising strategies to cease the disease process altogether (Campos & Fontana, 2022). Despite the acceptance of risk assessment as part of modern methodologies in the prevention and management of caries leading to a more cost-effective approach, a significant number of dental practitioners do not appear to have adopted such strategies (Campos & Fontana, 2022). This lack of adoption may be attributed to the involvement of expert-based, subjective and unsatisfactorily validated tools to provide a proper classification of risk assessment (Fontana & Gonzalez-Cabezas, 2012).

In light of the fact that patients with SHCNs require individualised treatment plans due to the myriad of factors determining their condition, it might seem logical to advocate the involvement of caries risk assessment in the management of such individuals. Tools such as the ones by the American Dental Association (ADA), American Association of Pediatric Dentistry (AAPD) and Caries Management by Risk Assessment may be utilised (Campos & Fontana, 2022).

Further, questionnaires for caries risk assessment are easy to answer and provide an indication of the patient's medical and dental history, diet, access to care and oral hygiene habits (Campos & Fontana, 2022). People with cognitive impairment and young patients should undergo the assessment along with a care-giver/guardian/family-member. Such an assessment should include current and past experience of caries, frequency of carbohydrate consumption, plaque presence, being exposed to protective modalities such as fluorides and an assessment of a potential decrease in salivary flow (Fontana, 2015; Fontana et al., 2013).

A variety of risk factors may be involved which will depend on the type, level and number of disabilities of an individual. These might range from age, diet, oral hygiene and behaviour in children affected by autism spectrum disorders. Generally, a poor perception of behaviour has been observed to be related to having greater odds of dental needs being unmet (Campos & Fontana, 2022). At the other end of the age spectrum, frail adult and vulnerable elderly patients who are medically compromised may also be at an elevated caries risk, which often manifests as numerous lesions of an advanced nature involving the root surfaces of teeth and warrant prompt assessment and addressal due to their tendency for rapid progression (Fontana, 2015; Fontana et al., 2013).

Management of Caries in People with Disabilities

A systematic review in 2011, which concluded that more high-quality research was needed to form evidence to support the improvement of oral health in people with special needs, was a significant step in recognising an ignored aspect of oral health concern (Molina et al., 2011).

Even though caries prevalence may not be necessarily greater in individuals with disabilities when compared to those without disabilities, it has been reiterated a number of times that persons with disabilities have a greater number of lesions which are untreated and, hence, an increased unmet treatment need (Molina et al., 2022).

The management of carious lesions can be broadly divided into non-restorative/ preventive and restorative strategies and may further involve a combination of these. It has been suggested that the non-restorative treatment paradigm for carious lesions have been demonstrated to be effective, and these can be utilised with or without restorative procedures owing to their feasibility, safety and effectiveness (Slayton et al., 2018).

Non-restorative/Preventive Treatment

Evidence on caries management for the general population may be applicable to people with SHCNs due to a lack of specific evidence for the latter. Expert guidelines published in this regard stated that the utilisation of 5% sodium fluoride varnish, 38% silver diammine fluoride (SDF), 5000 ppm gel or toothpaste and 1.23% acidulated phosphate fluoride gel formed the most efficacious interventions (Slayton et al., 2018). It is also worthwhile to note that the same panel did not recommend the usage of 10% casein phosphopeptide amorphous calcium phosphate.

In children, the general population and people with SHCNs, sealants and fluorides have been evidenced to be effective preventive measures for the management of caries (Campos & Fontana, 2022). There is ample evidence in literature to support the ability of topical fluoride application in reducing the incidence of caries in both permanent and primary dentition including community water fluoridation as well as fluoride products (Campos & Fonatana, 2022).

Fluoride Toothpastes

Fluoride toothpastes are manufactured and made available in a variety of strengths with 1000 ppm fluoride content toothpastes being the most commonly available over-the-counter and those with a higher concentration necessitating a prescription. As the action of fluoride is typically considered to be dose-dependent, rinsing of toothpastes should be kept at a minimum to enhance the effect of fluoride application (Campos & Fontana, 2022).

Further issues that may arise with fluoridated toothpastes may be attributed to those of a sensory nature as a result of the texture, flavour or taste, as has been observed in people with autism spectrum disorders (Campos & Fontana, 2022). The decision of choosing the fluoride concentration of a toothpaste should be based upon the risk assessment for caries which may include fluoride exposure information pertaining to both professional application and as a result of self-care (Walsh et al., 2019). Risks such as those of fluoride toxicity and fluorosis as a result of dentifrice ingestion should also be considered (Walsh et al., 2019).

Toothbrushing

Plaque removal by mechanical methods commonly involves the utilisation of tooth-brushing with powered or manual toothbrushes and a fluoridated toothpaste, twice a day for two minutes (Walsh et al., 2019). For patients with SHCNs it is advisable to recommend supervised toothbrushing and educating care-givers in oral hygiene techniques along with recommending a higher frequency of recall visits (Campos & Fontana, 2022). For people with intellectual disabilities, however, these recommen-dations constitute evidence of low quality with the benefits being somewhat unclear (Walsh et al., 2019). Consideration must also be made of injuries which might occur during toothbrushing in patients with SHCNs.

Fluoride Rinses

Sodium fluoride rinses are another modality utilised to increase the exposure to fluoride to prevent carious lesions. These can be utilised in varying concentra-tions, with 900 ppm F recommended for weekly usage and 230 ppm F as part of a daily usage regime (Campos & Fontana, 2022). Sodium fluoride rinses can be utilised both at home and as part of school programmes. As a result of fluo-ride action being dose-dependent, increased exposure and higher concentration are recommended for in-office and at-home use in managing patients classified at a high risk of caries (Campos & Fontana, 2022). Other professional application products such as varnishes and gels may be administered at 3–6-month intervals for patients at a moderate risk for caries and particularly for those at a higher caries risk (Paris et al., 2020; Waldron et al., 2019).

Silver Diammine Fluoride

SDF has emerged relatively recently as a material which potentially modifies biofilm and promotes remineralisation. In the United States, SDF has approval from the Food and Drug Administration in the form of a professional desensitiser; however, there is evidence in literature to support its efficacy as an agent which arrests caries in both the permanent and primary dentition (Campos & Fontana, 2022). As such, SDF brings about an arrest of coronal carious lesions as well as those on the root surface, all the while being user-friendly, safe, efficacious and affordable (Campos & Fontana, 2022). It has been suggested that SDF utilises the antibacterial properties of silver as well as the effects of remineralisation exerted by fluoride (Mei et al., 2013, 2017). SDF has been recommended for utilisation in people with SHCNs, frail adults, vulnerable elderly and in young children (Gao et al., 2020).

The AAPD's recommendations in 2018 stated that 38% SDF application could be utilised in adolescents and children, including ones with SHCNs to arrest cavitated lesions (Campos & Fontana, 2022). The utilisation of SDF is particularly lucrative in people with SHCNs as the application process is straightforward and simple. It involves a SDF saturated microbrush for agent delivery in relative isolation. The patient is advised to avoid drinking and eating for half an hour post application. The treated area must be reassessed at a follow-up visit which can be a few weeks later. It has been noted that reapplication after 6 months improves the results, with caries arrest being evident upon hardening of the cavitated area. A significant drawback of SDF application is the dark staining that is observed within a few days or even hours of application which might dissuade its usage in areas of aesthetic concern.

Dental Sealants

Pit and fissure sealants are regarded as an acceptable caries prevention methodology. Sealants are generally placed between one to one and a half years post eruption owing to the enamel not being completely mature in this time frame (Morales-Chávez et al., 2014). Resin-based sealants were introduced in 1965 and upon placement, form a physical barrier which prevents the microorganisms in the pits and fissures from deriving nutrition from sources in the oral cavity (Morales-Chávez et al., 2014). Further, the application of this material necessitates strict isolation, which might be difficult to achieve in patients with SHCNs and lead to failure of the procedure.

Glass ionomers, introduced in 1974, tide over some of the issues faced with resin-based sealants (Morales-Chávez et al., 2014). This material has the property of releasing fluoride in its vicinity even up to a year after placement and has been suggested for utilisation in patients with SHCNs as they decrease caries occurrence and do not require strict isolation (Morales-Chávez et al., 2014). Glass ionomer sealants also require less time in application as they do not require acid etching as with resin-based sealants and hence are advantageous in people with SHCNs (Morales-Chávez et al., 2014).

Antimicrobials

Antimicrobials is another set of materials which have been studied in terms of their ability to contribute towards the management of carious lesions. Owing to their antimicrobial and non-cariogenic properties, regular use of polyol combinations or xylitol in lozenges and chewing gums has been suggested to form an adjunctive measure in the prevention of carious lesions in the coronal region and root surfaces (Campos & Fontana, 2022). Professional application of thymol/chlorhexidine varnish has been demonstrated to be efficacious in the prevention as well as arrest of root caries (Walsh et al., 2015; Navarro Azevedo de Azeredo et al., 2019).

Older individuals exhibit a particularly high risk of developing carious lesions especially on the root surfaces. This may be attributed to a variety of factors such as poor oral hygiene, exposure of root surfaces, medications which decrease salivary flow and a high frequency of sugar consumption (Campos & Fontana, 2022). The quarterly or even four times a year application of 5% sodium fluoride varnish has been demonstrated to decrease caries in older people under institutional care (Innes & Evans, 2009). Another effective measure that has been investigated is the combination of oral health education, 38% SDF and 5000 ppm F toothpaste utilisation biannually which has demonstrated efficacy in arresting carious lesions on root surfaces (Campos & Fontana, 2022).

Restorative Treatment

Minimally invasive procedures are accepted as best practice in controlling and managing caries as well as in preserving natural teeth and hard tissues (Marchini et al., 2019). The priority of restorative treatment must focus on preserving healthy dental structures, remineralisation and obtaining margins conducive for an appropriate restorative seal (Marchini et al., 2019). The pulpal stress should be minimised with the aim being to enhance restorative success as much as possible and prolonging the life of the tooth. As part of this concept, it is not necessary to remove demineralised or infected tissue in its entirety and carious tissue should ideally be removed only enough to form a good restorative seal (Marchini et al., 2019). In deep carious lesions in the vicinity of the pulp, selective soft dentin removal has been demonstrated to be successful while, in shallow lesions away from the pulpal tissue, selective firm dentin removal may be executed (Schwendicke et al., 2016).

Different restorative materials have been studied over the years. Amalgam was long considered a successful restorative material owing to its antimicrobial properties and longevity (Schwendicke et al., 2016). It has, however, fallen largely into disuse due to environmental and aesthetic concerns (Marchini et al., 2019).

The phasing out of amalgam has witnessed the emergence of composites as a worthwhile replacement. Though the longevity of these materials competes with that of amalgam, they are more susceptible to the occurrence of secondary caries particularly in patients at high risk (Marchini et al., 2019).

Earlier regarded as a temporary restorative material, the high-viscosity glass ionomer cements (GICs) improve upon longevity to bring them potentially at par with composites and amalgam (Schwendicke et al., 2016). GICs have the property for adhesion to both dentin and enamel as well as fluoride release and biocompatibility. They do not require strict moisture control in their application, and this along with the property of dentin and enamel adherence contributes to them being less technique-sensitive and easily utilisable in patients with SHCNs.

Atraumatic Restorative Treatment (ART)

ART involves manual excavation of soft carious lesions with subsequent restoration with GIC (high viscosity) (Marchini et al., 2019). Art has been successfully utilised in people with SHCNs and frail adults due to its simplicity which reduces patient discomfort and anxiety (Marchini et al., 2019). ART has demonstrated utility in settings outside the dental office, exhibits longevity comparable to conventional restorations, has satisfactory patient acceptance and is cost-effective (da Mata et al., 2014; da Mata et al., 2015a, b).

Patient Management

Patients with special needs may present with significant challenges during the treatment procedure. Patients exhibiting aggressive behavioural patterns may cause harm to the dental team, care-givers or to themselves (Marchini et al., 2019). This behaviour may manifest in varying forms such as physical forms of aggression, inability/ refusal to follow instructions and inability to comprehend the procedure (Marchini et al., 2019). Certain elementary communication strategies must be employed by the dental team rendering care. These include a gentle, respectful and patient approach, maintaining eye contact, avoiding sudden or fast movements, introducing oneself, addressing the patient by their name, inserting positive reinforcement, explaining the procedure in plain language and repeating these if necessary (Marchini et al., 2019).

Patients with SHCNs may present with multiple conditions, impairments and comorbidities. This makes it essential to evaluate such individuals with a multidisciplinary approach and provide patients and care-givers with information about the examination, treatment plan and instructions regarding oral hygiene maintenance (Marchini et al., 2017).

The practitioner must realise that the care of such individuals may involve a number of people, and the perspectives and expectations of each individual must be considered to enhance the long-term success of treatment (Marchini et al., 2019). Ideally, a multidisciplinary conference regarding the patient's condition must be undertaken but seldom happens except in certain institutional models (Marchini et al., 2019). It is important to consider communication with the patient's care-giver/ guardian in cases of obtaining consent and also take note of the fact that some patients may have different individuals responsible for their health and finances (Marchini et al., 2019).

Conclusion

Just as it is in the general population, dental caries continues to have a significant burden upon people living with disabilities. Such individuals have been identified to demonstrate a greater number of untreated carious lesions which signifies a massive unmet treatment need. Such a presentation may be attributed to the variety and severity of disabilities and medical conditions that such individuals face which includes social and financial barriers to accessing care. Management of dental caries should preferably involve a preventive or non-restorative approach and even in cases where restorative treatment inevitably needs to be rendered, the procedure should be as minimally invasive as possible. The restorative techniques and materials employed should be chosen to be conducive towards the unique conditions of the patient so as to enhance outcomes. Patient behaviour management and taking the guardian/care-givers into confidence as well as employing a multidisciplinary pattern of care and conference may aid in improving the long-term treatment outcomes for individuals living with disabilities.

References

Campos, M. S., & Fontana, M. (2022). Caries Management in Special Care Dentistry. Dental clinics of North America, 66(2), 169–179. https://doi.org/10.1016/j.cden.2021.12.003.

da Mata, C., Allen, P. F., Cronin, M., O'Mahony, D., McKenna, G., & Woods, N. (2014). Cost-effectiveness of ART restorations in elderly adults: A randomized clinical trial. Community Dentistry and Oral Epidemiology, 42(1), 79–87.

da Mata, C., Allen, P. F., McKenna, G., Cronin, M., O'Mahony, D., & Woods, N. (2015a). Two-year survival of ART restorations placed in elderly patients: A randomised controlled clinical trial. Journal of Dentistry, 43(4), 405–411. https://doi.org/10.1016/j.jdent.2015.01.003.

da Mata, C., Cronin, M., O'Mahony, D., McKenna, G., Woods, N., & Allen, P. F. (2015b). Subjective impact of minimally invasive dentistry in the oral health of older patients. Clinical Oral Investigations, 19(3), 681–687. https://doi.org/10.1007/s00784-014-1290-6.

Fontana, M. (2015). The clinical, environmental, and behavioral factors that foster early childhood caries: Evidence for caries risk assessment. Pediatric Dentistry, 37(3), 217–225.

Fontana, M., & Gonzalez-Cabezas, C. (2012). Minimal intervention dentistry: part 2. Caries risk assessment in adults. *British Dental Journal, 213*(9), 447–451. https://doi.org/10.1038/sj.bdj. 2012.1008.

Fontana, M., Cabezas, C. G., & Fitzgerald, M. (2013). Cariology for the 21st century. *The Journal of the Michigan Dental Association, 4*, 32–40.

Gao, S. S., Chen, K. J., Duangthip, D., Wong, M. C. M., Lo, E. C. M., & Chu, C. H. (2020). Arresting early childhood caries using silver and fluoride products-a randomised trial. *Journal of Dentistry, 103*, 103522. https://doi.org/10.1016/j.jdent.2020.103522.

Innes, N., & Evans, D. (2009). Managing dental caries in children: Improving acceptability and outcomes through changing priorities and understanding the disease. *British dental journal, 206*(10), 549–550. https://doi.org/10.1038/sj.bdj.2009.471.

Khalid, I., Chandrupatla, S. G., Kaye, E., Scott, T., & Sohn, W. (2019). Dental sealant prevalence among children with special health care needs: National health and nutrition examination survey (NHANES) 2013 to 2014. *Pediatric Dentistry, 41*(3), 186–190.

Marchini, L., Ettinger, R., & Hartshorn, J. (2019). Personalized dental caries management for frail older adults and persons with special needs. *Dental Clinics of North America, 63*(4), 631–651. https://doi.org/10.1016/j.cden.2019.06.003.

Marchini, L., Hartshorn, J. E., Cowen, H., Dawson, D. V., & Johnsen, D. C. (2017). A teaching tool for establishing risk of oral health deterioration in elderly patients: development, implementation, and evaluation at a U.S. Dental School. *Journal of Dental Education, 81*(11), 1283–1290. https://doi.org/10.21815/JDE.017.086.

Mei, M. L., Chu, C. H., Low, K. H., Che, C. M., & Lo, E. C. (2013). Caries arresting effect of silver diamine fluoride on dentine carious lesion with S. mutans and L. acidophilus dual-species cariogenic biofilm. *Medicina oral, patologia oral y cirugia bucal, 18*(6), e824–e831. https://doi.org/10.4317/medoral.18831.

Mei, M. L., Nudelman, F., Marzec, B., Walker, J. M., Lo, E. C. M., Walls, A. W., & Chu, C. H. (2017). Formation of fluorohydroxyapatite with silver diamine fluoride. *Journal of Dental Research, 96*(10), 1122–1128. https://doi.org/10.1177/0022034517709738.

Molina, G. F., Leal, S. C., & Frencken, J. E. (2011). Strategies for managing carious lesions in patients with disabilities—A systematic review. *Journal of Disability and Oral Health, 12*(4), 159.

Molina, G., Zar, M., Dougall, A., & McGrath, C. (2022). Management of dental caries lesions in patients with disabilities: Update of a systematic review. *Frontiers in Oral Health, 3*, 980048.

Morales-Chávez, M. C., & Nualart-Grollmus, Z. C. (2014). Retention of a resin-based sealant and a glass ionomer used as a fissure sealant in children with special needs. *Journal of Clinical and Experimental Dentistry, 6*(5), e551–e555. https://doi.org/10.4317/jced.51688.

Navarro Azevedo de Azeredo, F., Silva Guimarães, L., Azeredo A Antunes, L., & Santos Antunes, L. (2019). Global prevalence of dental caries in athletes with intellectual disabilities: An epidemiological systematic review and meta-analysis. *Special Care in Dentistry : Official Publication of the American Association of Hospital Dentists, the Academy of Dentistry for the Handicapped, and the American Society for Geriatric Dentistry, 39*(2), 114–124. https://doi.org/10.1111/scd. 12349.

Paris, S., Banerjee, A., Bottenberg, P., Breschi, L., Campus, G., Doméjean, S., Ekstrand, K., Giacaman, R. A., Haak, R., Hannig, M., Hickel, R., Juric, H., Lussi, A., Machiulskiene, V., Manton, D., Jablonski-Momeni, A., Santamaria, R., Schwendicke, F., Splieth, C. H., Tassery, H., Opdam, N. (2020). How to intervene in the caries process in older adults: A joint ORCA and EFCD expert delphi consensus statement. *Caries Research, 54*(5–6), 1–7. Advance online publication. https://doi.org/10.1159/000510843.

Pini, D. M., Fröhlich, P. C., & Rigo, L. (2016). Oral health evaluation in special needs individuals. *Einstein (Sao Paulo, Brazil), 14*(4), 501–507. https://doi.org/10.1590/S1679-45082016AO3712.

Robertson, M. D., Schwendicke, F., de Araujo, M. P., Radford, J. R., Harris, J. C., McGregor, S., & Innes, N. P. T. (2019). Dental caries experience, care index and restorative index in children with learning disabilities and children without learning disabilities; a systematic review and meta-analysis. *BMC Oral Health, 19*(1), 146. https://doi.org/10.1186/s12903-019-0795-4.

Schwendicke, F., Frencken, J. E., Bjorndal, L., et al. (2016). Managing carious lesions: Consensus recommendations on carious tissue removal. *Advances in Dental Research, 28*(2), 58–67.

Slayton, R. L., Urquhart, O., Araujo, M. W. B., Fontana, M., Guzmán-Armstrong, S., Nascimento, M. M., Nový, B. B., Tinanoff, N., Weyant, R. J., Wolff, M. S., Young, D. A., Zero, D. T., Tampi, M. P., Pilcher, L., Banfield, L., & Carrasco-Labra, A. (2018). Evidence-based clinical practice guideline on nonrestorative treatments for carious lesions: A report from the American Dental Association. *Journal of the American Dental Association (1939), 149*(10), 837–849.e19. https://doi.org/10.1016/j.adaj.2018.07.002.

Waldron, C., Nunn, J., Mac Giolla Phadraig, C., Comiskey, C., Guerin, S., van Harten, M. T., Donnelly-Swift, E., & Clarke, M. J. (2019). Oral hygiene interventions for people with intellectual disabilities. *The Cochrane Database of Systematic Reviews, 5*(5), CD012628. https://doi.org/10.1002/14651858.CD012628.pub2.

Walsh, T., Oliveira-Neto, J. M., & Moore, D. (2015). Chlorhexidine treatment for the prevention of dental caries in children and adolescents. *The Cochrane Database of Systematic Reviews, 2015*(4), CD008457.

Walsh, T., Worthington, H. V., Glenny, A. M., Marinho, V. C., & Jeroncic, A. (2019). Fluoride toothpastes of different concentrations for preventing dental caries. *The Cochrane Database of Systematic Reviews, 3*(3), CD007868. https://doi.org/10.1002/14651858.CD007868.pub3.

Dental Trauma and Disability

Abstract People living with disabilities may be particularly prone to incurring dental trauma as is the case in those with issues surrounding neuromuscular coordination. Dental trauma may affect both primary and permanent dentition across age groups. This is of significance since the management of such presentations changes depending upon the type of dentition affected and its stage of development, amongst other factors. Patients and care-givers in particular should be aware of any emergency measures they can undertake along with information regarding what should not be done in case a tooth is knocked out. Practitioners should be aware of strategies they can employ to effectively deal with such cases without compromising on the standard of care.

Keywords Dental trauma · Traumatic dental injuries · Disability · Special needs

Dental trauma or Traumatic Dental Injuries (TDIs) have been reported in the general population amongst children and adolescents. The reported prevalence has ranged from 7.3 to 58.6% (Ferreira et al., 2011). By comparison, there are fewer reports in literature describing the prevalence of TDIs in people with SHCNs (Ferreira et al., 2011). In those with handicaps, the prevalence has been reported to be 28.8 and 18% in two separate studies (Nunn & Murray, 1987; Ohito et al., 1992).

Three studies have reported the prevalence of TDIs in people with cerebral palsy to be 57 and 10.6%, with those attending a rehabilitation centre for severe forms of physical impairment having a reported TDI prevalence of 20% (Costa et al., 2008; dos Santos & Souza, 2009; Holan et al., 2005). Individuals with sensory impairment have a reported prevalence of dental trauma of 9% with those having a hearing impairment reporting an 11.4% prevalence of TDIs (AlSarheed et al., 2003).

TDIs can potentially impact the emotional, social and psychological well-being of people. Conditions affecting the balance, coordination, safety reflexes and responsiveness of individuals can lead to an uptick in TDI incidence (Devi et al., 2024). In general, it is acknowledged that conditions such as cerebral palsy, epilepsy, attention deficit hyperactivity disorder and autism, which affect neuromuscular coordination tend to increase people's chances of injury (Devi et al., 2024). Further, children with

V. Sahni, *Oral Health in People with Disabilities*,
SpringerBriefs in Modern Perspectives on Disability Research,
https://doi.org/10.1007/978-981-96-2779-0_5

SHCNs such as those with impaired motor coordination, involuntary movements, intellectual disability, masticatory muscle spasticity and pathological oral reflexes have been identified to exhibit a greater prevalence of dental trauma (Al-Batayneh et al., 2017).

It can thus be acknowledged that even though individuals with SHCNs are at a greater risk of undergoing TDIs, the type of disability may also be of importance in determining outcomes. Over a period of time, people with SHCNs have found a greater integration into society with encouragement being made to participate in various social activities and sports events which may further increase the susceptibility to TDIs (Devi et al., 2024).

Patient Evaluation

History

A thorough history should be recorded which should include the number, type and severity of the disability along with any underlying medical conditions and comorbidities. The medical history should also include the status of tetanus immunisation, allergies and medications. The time, site and mode of injury should be recorded. The time from injury will provide an indicator of prognosis as well as guide management. Any associated injuries may be gleaned from the mode of injury. Prompt referrals should be made in case signs of neurological compromise are evident, such as headache, nausea, vomiting, unconsciousness, irritability, amnesia, dizziness and lethargy.

Examination

Extra-orally, the facial skeleton must be examined for discontinuities. The temporomandibular joints should be examined for any abnormalities along with a note being made of any extra-oral bruises or wounds. The cervical spine should be examined, and any abnormality should prompt a referral. Intra-oral soft tissues such as the oral mucosa, gingivae, tongue, palate and frenae should be examined. Anterior and posterior dentition should be thoroughly examined to check for increased mobility, change in position or colour, fractures, pulpal exposure, pain, sensitivity and change in occlusion.

Radiography

Radiographs aid the clinician in evaluating unerupted dentition, root development, peri-apical condition, fractures, root resorption, pulp chamber size, changes in tooth position and foreign bodies/dental fragments. Any radiography must take into account the patient's comfort in positioning and if necessitated, alternatives to intra-oral radiography such as panoramic views and three-dimensional alternatives may be considered. Baseline radiographs are useful in providing a benchmark for future comparison to monitor progress. A number of pathological changes may not be apparent in the immediate term after injury and may manifest at a later point in time.

Types of Dentoalveolar Injuries

Fractures of the crown and root of the dentition may result as a consequence of trauma. Fractures of the crown can be described as either uncomplicated (i.e. involving the enamel and dentin or the enamel alone) or complicated (i.e. involves the pulpal tissue) (McTigue 2012). Root fractures can be oblique, vertical or horizontal (McTigue 2012).

Luxation injuries involve the supporting apparatus of the dentition including the alveolar bone and periodontal ligament (PDL). These injuries can be further classi-fied into different types. A *concussion* involves a tooth which may have tenderness upon bite pressure and is neither displaced nor loose (McTigue 2012). *Subluxation* involves a loose tooth which is in its socket (McTigue 2012). *Extrusion* is when the tooth has undergone a central dislocation from the socket (McTigue 2012). *Intrusion* involves the tooth being displaced apically from the socket. *Lateral luxation* denotes a displacement of the tooth in a lateral, posterior or anterior dimension (McTigue 2012). *Avulsion* is when the tooth is displaced in its entirety from the socket.

Dos Santos et al. reported that the maxillary central incisors of both the permanent and primary dentition were most often involved in people with cerebral palsy as well as those without it (dos Santos & Souza, 2009). They also found that in their group of cerebral palsy patients, fractures of the enamel and dentin and that of the enamel alone, without pulpal involvement, were the most common form of TDI.

Oliveira et al. also reported that the anterior dentition was most commonly affected by trauma which may be attributed to the greater proclination of maxillary central incisors as compared to their mandibular counterparts which positions the former to be the first to receive a traumatic blow (Oliveira et al., 2007). Additionally, the authors also stated that the maxilla being fixed is unable to move and reduce impact forces in contrast to the mandible, and this may contribute to a greater incidence of TDIs in the upper jaw (Oliveira et al., 2007).

Treatment of Traumatic Dental Injuries

Primary Dentition

The main goal of managing injuries to the primary dentition is preserving the developing successional dentition. Care-giver, parents and patients should be informed of the relationship between the primary and permanent dentition. The approach should be thorough and empathetic. It should aim to take into confidence everyone involved in the care of the person with SHCNs. It is imperative to ensure an understanding is reached upon the treatment plan and its rationale not only to enhance long-term outcomes but also for the purposes of consent.

Enamel Fracture

Any sharp edges should be smoothened. The patient/parent/care-giver should be advised to be careful while eating to avoid further traumatising the tooth. Oral hygiene should be maintained in the area of concern with a cotton swab or soft brush with 0.1–0.2% chlorhexidine gluconate mouthwash two times a day for a week (Day et al., 2020).

Uncomplicated Enamel-Dentin Fracture

Composite or glass ionomer should be utilised to provide coverage for any dentin that has been exposed. Restoration of lost tooth structure can be done with composite in the immediate term or later as well (Day et al., 2020). Oral hygiene and re-traumatisation care should be followed as for enamel fractures.

Complicated Crown Fracture

Pulp preservation by means of a partial pulpotomy must be undertaken under local anaesthesia. For large exposures of the pulp, a cervical pulpotomy is the indication (Day et al., 2020). The treatment must be rendered bearing in mind the patient's capacity to tolerate an invasive procedure in light of the potential dental anxiety it may induce in the long term (Day et al., 2020). Oral hygiene and re-traumatisation care as usual are to be recommended.

Crown Root Fracture

In an emergency situation, no treatment may be rendered if a prompt specialist referral can be made (Day et al., 2020). If the tooth is restorable, the loose fragment should be removed and restoration should follow with or without pulpal treatment depending on whether an exposure occurred (Day et al., 2020). In case the tooth is unrestorable, the loose fragments must be removed or the entire tooth may be extracted (Day et al., 2020). Usual re-traumatisation and oral hygiene measures are recommended.

Root Fracture

In case of an undisplaced coronal fragment, no treatment is necessary (Day et al., 2020). In case of a displaced coronal fragment which is not overly mobile, the fragment can be allowed to reposition spontaneously even in the presence of a certain amount of occlusal interference (Day et al., 2020). In case the displaced coronal fragment is overly mobile and causes occlusal interference as well then either the loose fragment can be extracted under local anaesthesia while the apical part is left to resorb *or* the loose fragment can be repositioned and any instability can be stabilised for four weeks with a flexible splint (Day et al., 2020). Usual re-traumatisation and oral hygiene measures are recommended.

Alveolar Fracture

Any fragment which is displaced and mobile or interferes with the occlusion needs to be repositioned under local anaesthesia (Day et al., 2020). The segment should be stabilised for four weeks with a flexible splint (Day et al., 2020). Usual re-traumatisation and oral hygiene measures are recommended.

Concussion and Subluxation

No treatment is necessitated and the tooth should be observed with the usual re-traumatisation and oral hygiene measures being recommended.

Extrusive Luxation

The treatment plan is determined by the mobility, displacement, stage of root formation, occlusal interference and the patient's capacity to tolerate treatment (Day et al., 2020). The tooth can be left to reposition spontaneously if it does not cause occlusal interference (Day et al., 2020). In cases where the tooth is extruded beyond 3 mm or exhibits excessive mobility, it should be extracted under local anaesthesia (Day et al., 2020). Usual re-traumatisation and oral hygiene measures are recommended.

Lateral Luxation

In cases of no or minimal interference with occlusion, the tooth can be allowed to reposition spontaneously, which usually happens within a six-month time frame (Day et al., 2020). Where the tooth has undergone a severe displacement, it can be extracted under local anaesthesia in case it poses an aspiration or ingestion risk; alternatively, the tooth can be repositioned and stabilised for four weeks with a flexible splint (Day et al., 2020). Usual re-traumatisation and oral hygiene measures are recommended.

Intrusive Luxation

Regardless of the direction of displacement, the tooth should be allowed to reposition spontaneously which can happen within 6 months to a year (Day et al., 2020). Usual re-traumatisation and oral hygiene measures are recommended.

Avulsion

It is not advisable to replant avulsed primary dentition. Usual re-traumatisation and oral hygiene measures are recommended.

Permanent Dentition

Enamel Infraction

This type of injury constitutes a craze/crack/incomplete breach in the enamel without losing any tooth structure. Generally no treatment is necessary unless the infraction is severe, in which case sealing with bonding resin must be performed to avoid microbial contamination and discoloration (Bourguignon et al., 2020).

Uncomplicated Crown Fracture (Enamel Only)

In case of availability of the tooth fragment, it can be bonded to the tooth (Bour-guignon et al., 2020). Otherwise, the edges of the tooth can be smoothened or a composite restoration can be placed (Bourguignon et al., 2020).

Uncomplicated Crown Fracture (Enamel and Dentin)

In case of availability of the tooth fragment, it should first be soaked in saline or water for twenty minutes to undergo rehydration before being bonded to the tooth (Bourguignon et al., 2020). Exposed dentin should be covered with composite resin and bonding agent or with glass ionomer (Bourguignon et al., 2020). In cases where the dentin is in the vicinity of the pulp, a lining of calcium hydroxide should be placed followed by glass ionomer (Bourguignon et al., 2020).

Uncomplicated Crown Fracture (Crown and Root in the Absence of Pulp Exposure)

A temporary stabilisation of the loose fragment may be attempted till a definitive course of action is decided (Bourguignon et al., 2020). The mobile or coronal fragment may be removed and a restoration may be considered (Bourguignon et al., 2020). Exposed dentin can be covered with composite resin and a bonding agent or with glass ionomer (Bourguignon et al., 2020). Future treatment may include surgical or orthodontic extrusion, root submergence, endodontic therapy, extraction, intentional replantation and autotransplantation (Bourguignon et al., 2020).

Complicated Crown Fracture (Enamel and Dentin with Pulp Exposure)

Pulp capping or partial pulpotomy are recommended in cases where the apices are open or in immature roots (Bourguignon et al., 2020). In cases where the root has completed development, conservative forms of pulp treatment are preferred (Bourguignon et al., 2020).

Complicated Crown Fracture (Crown and Root with Pulp Exposure)

Temporary stabilisation of the tooth must be done till a definitive treatment plan is executed. Pulp preservation should be done for immature teeth, and pulpectomy is indicated for mature dentition (Bourguignon et al., 2020). Future treatment options may include endodontic and restorative therapy, surgical or orthodontic extrusion, extraction, root submergence and autotransplantation (Bourguignon et al., 2020).

Root Fracture

A coronal fragment, if displaced, should be repositioned promptly with a confirmatory radiograph to ascertain this (Bourguignon et al., 2020). The segment can be stabilised for four weeks using a flexible splint, and cervical fractures may require a longer splinting time of four months (Bourguignon et al., 2020). The coronal fragment in cervical fractures should not be removed at the time of an emergency visit since these injuries can heal (Bourguignon et al., 2020). It is not advisable to commence endodontic therapy at the time of the emergency visit (Bourguignon et al., 2020). It is recommended to monitor fracture healing for up to a year at least along with the pulp status of the tooth as well (Bourguignon et al., 2020). The coronal segment may exhibit infection and pulpal necrosis at a later stage which may necessitate endodontic therapy of this segment alone along with apexification (Bourguignon et al., 2020). In cases of mature dentition where the fracture line is present above the crest of the alveolar bone, a mobile coronal fragment can be removed, followed by endodontic therapy and a post-retained restoration (Bourguignon et al., 2020).

Alveolar Fracture

The displaced fragment should be repositioned and splinted for four weeks with a flexible splint (Bourguignon et al., 2020). The pulpal status of the affected dentition must be monitored at regular intervals.

Concussion

It does not necessitate any treatment; however, the pulpal status should be monitored for a year at least (Bourguignon et al., 2020).

Subluxation

Generally no treatment is required unless the tooth is overly mobile or tender upon biting, in which case, it should be stabilised for a period of up to two weeks with a flexible splint (Bourguignon et al., 2020). Regular pulpal status monitoring must be done for a year at least.

Extrusive Luxation

Tooth should be repositioned under local anaesthesia and stabilised with a flexible splint for two weeks (Bourguignon et al., 2020). In case a fracture has occurred with respect to the marginal bone, an additional four weeks of splinting is recommended (Bourguignon et al., 2020). Pulpal status monitoring in advised along with the institution of endodontic therapy if indicated.

Lateral Luxation

The tooth should be repositioned under local anaesthesia and further stabilised with a flexible splint for four weeks (Bourguignon et al., 2020). Further treatment is based upon subsequent pulpal status monitoring and endodontics evaluation two weeks after injury (Bourguignon et al., 2020).

Intrusive Luxation

For teeth with an immature root, if no spontaneous re-eruption occurs within four weeks then repositioning by orthodontic means should be initiated along with pulpal status monitoring (Bourguignon et al., 2020). In cases where the pulp becomes infected and necrotic or exhibits signs of inflammation, endodontic therapy should be considered (Bourguignon et al., 2020). The care-givers/parents/guardian should be explained the necessity and importance of follow-ups.

Teeth with mature roots should be allowed an opportunity to re-erupt in cases where the intrusion is less than 3 mm (Bourguignon et al., 2020). If the tooth does not re-erupt within a span of 8 weeks, it should be stabilised with a flexible splint for 4 weeks or orthodontically repositioned to avoid ankylosis (Bourguignon et al., 2020). For cases of intrusion in the range of 3–7 mm or beyond, it is preferable to perform a surgical repositioning over an orthodontic one (Bourguignon et al., 2020). As is quite often the case, in dentition with completed root formation, pulpal necrosis ensues which needs the institution of endodontic therapy at two weeks or whenever the tooth position is amenable for the same (Bourguignon et al., 2020).

Avulsion

The survival of avulsed permanent dentition is dependent upon the time elapsed out of the socket (McTigue 2012). The maintenance of PDL vitality is imperative with greater than 90% of such teeth exhibiting survival if they are replanted in under five minutes (McTigue 2012). In cases where the out of socket time in a dry environment exceeds an hour, the chances of survival become near zero (McTigue 2012). So it is important to stress that avulsed permanent dentition should be replanted at the earliest by the first person who is capable of doing so (McTigue 2012).

In order to replant the tooth, it should be held by the crown alone to avoid PDL damage. Then, the tooth should be gently rinsed in tap water or saline to remove debris which is followed by manual replantation of the tooth (McTigue 2012). The tooth should be stabilised for two weeks with a functional splint with a calcium hydroxide pulpectomy being completed after a week (McTigue 2012).

Since it is not always possible to immediately replant a tooth, the PDL vitality needs to be maintained by storage in media such as Hanks Balanced Salt Solution (HBSS) which acts by maintaining osmotic pressure and physiological pH (McTigue 2012). If HBSS is not available, cold milk is a suitable alternative and is also usually readily available, relatively aseptic and has an osmolality more conducive to PDL vitality as compared to tap water or saline (McTigue 2012).

Conclusion

There is evidence in literature to suggest that people with disabilities tend to exhibit a greater prevalence of TDIs as compared to the general population. In line with what is observed in people without disabilities, TDIs occur most commonly in the upper jaw and affect the front teeth most often. TDIs can involve both primary and permanent dentition which changes the management paradigm of the condition. It is important to take into account the unique condition of the patient and their disability in order to devise a treatment plan. Parents and care-givers should be made part of the treatment and follow-up process in order to enhance long-term outcomes. Information about emergency TDIs where time is of the essence, such as in avulsions, should be disseminated to the public so as to improve treatment outcomes. Prompt management, adequate referral and diligent follow-up can aid in improving long-term results.

References

Al-Batayneh, O. B., Owais, A. I., Al-Saydali, M. O., & Waldman, H. B. (2017). Traumatic dental injuries in children with special health care needs. *Dental Traumatology, 33*(4), 269–275.

AlSarheed, M., Bedi, R., & Hunt, N. P. (2003). Traumatised permanent teeth in 11–16-year-old Saudi Arabian children with a sensory impairment attending special schools. *Dental Traumatology : Official Publication of International Association for Dental Traumatology, 19*(3), 123–125. https://doi.org/10.1034/j.1600-9657.2003.00104.x.

Bourguignon, C., Cohenca, N., Lauridsen, E., Flores, M. T., O'Connell, A. C., Day, P. F., & Levin, L. (2020). International association of dental traumatology guidelines for the management of traumatic dental injuries: 1. Fractures and luxations. *Dental Traumatology, 36*(4), 314–330.

Costa, M. M., Afonso, R. L., Ruviére, D. B., & Aguiar, S. M. (2008). Prevalence of dental trauma in patients with cerebral palsy. *Special Care in Dentistry : Official Publication of the American Association of Hospital Dentists, the Academy of Dentistry for the Handicapped, and the American Society for Geriatric Dentistry, 28*(2), 61–64. https://doi.org/10.1111/j.1754-4505.2008.00013.x.

Day, P. F., Flores, M. T., O'Connell, A. C., Abbott, P. V., Tsilingaridis, G., Fouad, A. F., ... & Levin, L. (2020). International association of dental traumatology guidelines for the management of traumatic dental injuries: 3. Injuries in the primary dentition. *Dental Traumatology, 36*(4), 343–359.

Devi K. P., Tewari, N., O'Connell, A., Srivastav, S., Rajeswary, A., Upadhyay, A. D., & Bansal, K. (2024). Risk factors associated with traumatic dental injuries in individuals with special healthcare needs—a systematic review and meta-analysis. *Dental Traumatology, 40*(1), 91–110.

dos Santos, M. T., & Souza, C. B. (2009). Traumatic dental injuries in individuals with cerebral palsy. *Dental Traumatology: Official Publication of International Association for Dental Traumatology, 25*(3), 290–294. https://doi.org/10.1111/j.1600-9657.2009.00765.x.

Ferreira, M. C. D., Guare, R. O., Prokopowitsch, I., & Santos, M. T. B. R. (2011). Prevalence of dental trauma in individuals with special needs. *Dental Traumatology, 27*(2), 113–116.

Holan, G., Peretz, B., Efrat, J., & Shapira, Y. (2005). Traumatic injuries to the teeth in young individuals with cerebral palsy. *Dental Traumatology: Official Publication of International Association for Dental Traumatology, 21*(2), 65–69. https://doi.org/10.1111/j.1600-9657.2004.00274.x.

McTigue, D. J. (2012). Overview of trauma management for primary and young permanent teeth. *Dental Clinics of North America*, 39–57.

Nunn, J. H., & Murray, J. J. (1987). The dental health of handicapped children in Newcastle and Northumberland. *British Dental Journal, 162*(1), 9–14. https://doi.org/10.1038/sj.bdj.4806011.

Ohito, F. A., Opinya, G. N., & Wang'ombe, J. (1992). Traumatic dental injuries in normal and handicapped children in Nairobi, Kenya. *East African Medical Journal, 69*(12), 680–682.

Oliveira, L. B., Marcenes, W., Ardenghi, T. M., Sheiham, A., & Bönecker, M. (2007). Traumatic dental injuries and associated factors among Brazilian preschool children. *Dental Traumatology, 23*(2), 76–81.

Rodrigues, B., dos Santos, M. T., & Souza, C. B. C. (2009). Traumatic dental injuries in individuals with cerebral palsy. *Dental Traumatology, 25*(3), 290–294.

Malocclusion and Disability

Abstract Malocclusion can lead to compromised oral function and stability along with the indirect effect of detracting from one's appearance. These factors, in turn, might affect an individual's social acceptability and integration. Despite having serious consequences to living with a malocclusion, orthodontic treatment is still considered elective. This can be attributed to the significant management challenges posed by individuals with disabilities to the treatment process. Orthodontic treatment may tend to be prolonged and requires a long-term commitment on part of the patient and parent. It also requires a proficient and experienced specialist to manage such cases for which they might not have been specifically trained. However, if patient and parent cooperation can be achieved, a skilled practitioner may be able to undertake such a treatment by adapting it to the needs of the individual patient and can aim to achieve reasonable outcomes.

Keywords Malocclusion · Orthodontic treatment · Special needs · Disability

Introduction

It is generally acknowledged that people with disabilities tend to have worse oral health outcomes as compared to those without disabilities. Oral health is related to the overall health of an individual which is related to one's oral functions, communication abilities, appearance and quality of life. Individuals with disabilities may indulge in behaviours harmful to their oral health, may face challenges in accessing care and maintaining oral hygiene (Winter et al., 2008). Behaviours with an adverse impact on the oral health of people with disabilities include tongue thrusting, lip biting, ones which are mastication-related such as food pocketing, excessive amounts of swallowing, drooling and bruxism, and finger sucking (Winter et al., 2008).

Malocclusion (MO) is one of the most widely encountered oral issues, which can assume greater relevance in people with Special Healthcare Needs (SHCNs) as compared to the general population (Cabrita et al., 2017). As MO affects both aesthetics and function, it creates a hindrance in the social acceptability and integration of people with SHCNs who have been evidenced to exhibit a high MO prevalence (Cabrita et al., 2017). MO can cause phonetic difficulties as well as issues with swallowing and chewing (Cabrita et al., 2017).

Stomatognathic system parafunction and oral dysfunctions have been identified as the factors responsible for an increased prevalence of MO in children living with learning disabilities (Utomi & Onyeaso, 2009). Other factors such as abnormal habits, anomalous growth patterns and poor muscle coordination have also been suggested (Cabrita et al., 2017).

Prevalence

MO prevalence has been reported to be higher in people with disabilities (48–86%) in comparison to those without them (43.9–55.8%) (Brown & Schodel, 1976). An uptick in Class III malocclusion has been noted in concordance with a decrease in cases of Class II malocclusion in Down's syndrome (DS) patients when compared to controls (Brown & Schodel, 1976). Vittek et al. also reported similar results with 36.5% of DS patients with Class III and 9.8% with Class II malocclusion (Vittek et al., 1994).

DS has been suggested as a risk factor of significance for severe types of malocclusion (Shyama et al., 2001). This along with an elevated Class III malocclusion incidence in DS patients is attributable to an alteration in cranial-base relationships (Shyama et al., 2001).

Other factors such as reduced arch length, decreased arch size and diminished size of the maxilla, as is typical of DS, have also been suggested (Winter et al., 2008). Cerebral palsy (CP) patients also demonstrate an elevated treatment need for malocclusion. The most common type of malocclusion in CP patients has been evidenced to be Class II along with anterior diastema and missing dentition (Winter et al., 2008). This occurrence has been attributed to precocious primary teeth eruption along with head posture and an aberrant tongue (Winter et al., 2008). Excessive overjet in these patients has also been attributed to be the result of maxillary orbicularis failure and incompetence of the lips (Winter et al., 2008). It has been acknowledged that there is a variation in malocclusion depending upon the type of disability (mental or physical in origin) (Winter et al., 2008). People with intellectual disabilities have been observed to demonstrate a greater malocclusion prevalence in comparison to those with impairments in hearing or vision (Vignehsa et al., 1991; Oreland et al., 1987).

People with mental disability have been reported to score higher on the dental aesthetic index in comparison to those with general handicaps (Winter et al., 2008). In fact, the severity of the mental disability has been found to be associated with an increased incidence of hereditary and acquired orthodontic problems (Winter et al., 2008). In cleft patients, a Class III malocclusion has been attributed to surgical trauma as well as less than satisfactory primary palate development (Baek et al., 2002).

Necessity of Orthodontic Management

Even though the treatment need of patients with disabilities may be high, orthodontic intervention is regarded as an elective procedure (Becker et al., 2004). This is owed to the fact that such patients may not be completely cooperative and may face challenges such as routinely maintaining home care (Becker et al., 2004). This can further lead to issues involving periodontal disease and caries (Becker et al., 2004).

Challenges to Rendering Care

Patient behaviour may be potentially problematic as a result of an impaired ability to understand, reduced span of attention, limited ability to tolerate the procedure and elevated apprehension (Becker et al., 2004). Maintaining the patient in the dental chair may be a problem in light of uncontrolled movements and difficulty in sitting still (Becker et al., 2004). These patients may also have a significantly reduced level of cooperation, an exaggeration of the gag reflex and increased tendency to drool (Becker et al., 2004; Shapira et al., 1999). It has been reported that a greater proportion of parents presenting with their children having SHCNs for orthodontic treatment expected it to improve the child's oral function and health as well as their acceptance in society and quality of life (Becker et al., 2004).

Pre-treatment Visits

The general purpose of pre-treatment visits is to reduce the anxiety of the patient and make them feel comfortable and confident in the dental chair (Chaushu et al., 2012). It is also a useful opportunity to assess the patient's level of care being received at home and bring to the attention of the parent and patient where this may be improved (Chaushu et al., 2012). Parental participation should be encouraged and its benefits emphasised as a prerequisite for accepting the patient for treatment (Chaushu et al., 2012). A pre-treatment visit also provides an opportunity to evaluate the level of compliance and whether this might be maintainable throughout the course of treatment (Chaushu et al., 2012).

The patient and parent should be encouraged to maintain oral hygiene after debris and gingival inflammation have been pointed out. Asking the parent to take primary responsibility of toothbrushing and letting the child finish towards the end might be a good strategy as it involves the child and also familiarises them to foreign objects in the oral cavity (Chaushu et al., 2012). It is a reliable sign of compliance if the patient returns with good oral hygiene after being provided instruction for the same (Chaushu et al., 2012). The practitioner may choose to defer the treatment to a later date if oral care is lacking on part of the patient.

Behaviour Management

It must be acknowledged that patients with disabilities pose significant challenges to the treating orthodontist. Such patients have to be accepted with compassion and empathy in order to win their trust and indeed that of the parents/guardian/care-giver as well. Such patients necessitate longer chair-side time and more appointments (Becker et al., 2004). In cases where several procedures have to be performed under a single session of general anaesthesia (GA) or sedation, it is advisable to undertake these in a hospital setting (Becker et al., 2004).

At the same time, it is important to understand that negative behaviour patterns cannot be addressed with putting the patient under general anaesthesia for each visit (Chaushu et al., 2012). Pharmacological intervention may be required for anxious patients who are exacting, difficult and require nuanced biomechanics in protracted visits (Chaushu et al., 2012). Pharmacological assistance should be minimised and planned properly, which means that behaviour modification by the utilisation of techniques such as the 'tell-show-do' as well as negative and positive reinforcement assume greater significance (Chaushu et al., 2012). Pharmacological agents may be utilised via different routes such as oral (Valium, chloral hydrate, midazolam), trans-mucosal (nasal drops of midazolam), inhalation (nitrous oxide along with oxygen) and intravenous (propofol) (Chaushu et al., 2012). A combination of these pharmacological agents may be utilised to achieve the desired result and minimise side effects.

Treatment Challenges

The orthodontist must ensure that the care-giver/parent is completely on board with the treatment to be rendered and understands the kind of commitment it will require on their end (Rada et al., 2015). A substantial amount of time should be invested in having a discussion regarding the tolerance level of the patient in order to ensure that all parties are well aware and informed (Rada et al., 2015).

Parents or care-givers should assume the responsibility of maintaining oral hygiene since patients with intellectual and developmental disabilities have hyper-sensitive gag reflexes and impaired dexterity (Rada et al., 2015). It has been observed that for children living with their parents at home had the latter ensure responsibility for the child's daily care (Rada et al., 2015). However, for institutionalised children, the parents were not willing to assume direct responsibility or regularly visit the institution but were willing to teach and guide the attending staff (Becker et al., 2001).

Even though seizure history does not contraindicate treatment, seizure disorders which are poorly controlled preclude patients from undergoing orthodontic treatment (Rada et al., 2015). The occurrence of injury to soft tissues as a result of breakthrough seizures must be considered during the process of consent (Rada et al., 2015). Bands may be preferred in place of bonded brackets and might require a special order to the manufacturer (Rada et al., 2015). Bonded brackets may be dislodged in a number of patients with intellectual and developmental disabilities as a result of their forceful oral habits (Rada et al., 2015). The patients may demonstrate a lack of adaptive capacity for a number of appliances and alternative retention plans may need to be instituted (Rada et al., 2015). In general, the aim of the orthodontic treatment should be one of achieving an acceptable functional and aesthetic result (Rada et al., 2015).

Treatment Planning

The treatment plan is usually based on information gathered from the examination, radiography, photography, plaster casts and cephalometrics (Chaushu et al., 2012). For patients with SHCNs, if not managed properly, gathering this information can lead to negative experiences (Chaushu et al., 2012). Alternatively, obtaining diagnostic records can be deferred till the first session where sedation will be used, and a general treatment plan based on examination alone may be followed till then (Chaushu et al., 2012).

Orthodontic Treatment Adaptations

Regular orthodontic treatment may need to be adapted to suit the specific needs of patients with SHCNs.

Treatment Goals

Realistic treatment goals of achieving acceptable functional and aesthetic results should be maintained.

Records

Extra-oral radiography such as cephalograms and panoramic films are tolerated better than intra-oral radiography in the conscious patient, and the latter may need to be done under sedation (Chaushu et al., 2012). But even for extra-oral radiography it might be a challenge to hold the patient's head in position or maintain a particular posture, and it must be accepted that the diagnosis may have to be formulated with more focus on the findings of the examination (Chaushu et al., 2012).

Removable Appliances

Removable appliances are tolerated well with their placement being simple and learned easily (Chaushu et al., 2012). The activation and any adjustments are done outside the mouth which causes no disturbance to the patient's oral cavity by instruments or even the hands of the practitioner (Chaushu et al., 2012). Removable appliances are more conducive to the maintenance of oral hygiene, and it is recommended to use these to their fullest extent before moving on to fixed therapy (Chaushu et al., 2012). The construction and design of these appliances should involve a number of clasps for retention, so even patients with impaired dexterity who are intent on removing these might be able to adapt quickly (Chaushu et al., 2012).

Range of Appliance Action

Preference should be given to appliances which possess a long range of actions in order to keep inter-visit time as long as possible (Chaushu et al., 2012). A headgear cured into the acrylic of a removable plate has been found to be quite acceptable in such patients (Becker & Shapira, 1996; Becker et al., 2001). An appliance of this manner is easy to use, does not necessitate many visits for adjustment and is relatively safe (Chaushu et al., 2012). It also finds greater utility than elastics in managing space in cases where extractions are necessary (Chaushu et al., 2012).

Fixed Appliances

Once a Class I relationship has been achieved, the rest of the treatment can be accomplished with the help of a fixed appliance such as self-ligating systems or Tip-Edge Plus, which involve a minimal amount of frictional resistance in relation to sliding mechanics (Chaushu et al., 2012). Mechanics may further be simplified by considering non-routine extractions in patients with SHCNs even if this may not be the case for the general population (Chaushu et al., 2012).

Orthodontics and Sedation

The pharmacologic technique utilised should be the safest and simplest one available to accomplish the treatment to be performed. General anaesthesia and sedation should be considered only when the patient has admittedly failed to be conducive via behaviour management alone (Rada et al., 2015).

Conscious sedation may include oral sedatives, nitrous oxide and oxygen and/or intravenous agents. Minimal oral as well as nitrous oxide sedation can be undertaken by a single clinician; however, IV sedation requires a second clinician to administer the agents and for patient monitoring (Rada et al., 2015). Aspiration is a significant concern in patients undergoing sedation since the latter results in a total or partial loss of protective reflexes (Chaushu et al., 2012). In order to avoid bronchial infection or laryngospasm, it is imperative to prevent saliva, water, debris, blood or loose brackets from leaking into the airway (Chaushu et al., 2012).

Children with muscular dystrophy and CP are at a particularly increased risk given their diminished cough reflex (Chaushu et al., 2012). The dental assistant should be vigilant and make sure that no debris accumulates inside the mouth (Rada et al., 2015). Small objects may be ligated and a gauze throat screen can be utilised as measures against aspiration (Rada et al., 2015). The best method, however, might be the utilisation of a rubber dam, but this may not always be feasible, for example during band placement, taking impressions and soldered arch cementation (Chaushu et al., 2012). Indirect bonding has also been utilised to mitigate such a risk (Chaushu et al., 2012). Antisialogogue agents may be necessitated in order to effect moisture control as is necessary in certain procedures (Chaushu et al., 2012).

Treatment Relapse

Maintenance of a satisfactory result needs to be accomplished by placing a retainer for a protracted period of time (Chaushu et al., 2012). Patients with SHCNs demonstrated increased abnormalities in soft tissue behaviour, which includes an anomalous oral seal and tongue thrusting which are not usually conducive to treatment (Chaushu et al., 2012). This means that retention assumes greater significance in these patients as compared to the general population.

Treatment Failure

Generally treatment failure can be attributed to non-compliance with retention and may necessitate re-treatment (Chaushu et al., 2012). For this to be successful however, the patient and parent must assure the practitioner of a more disciplined compliance to retention (Chaushu et al., 2012). CP and myopathies can lead to vertical growth patterns only some of which may be controllable with active forms of retention (Chaushu et al., 2012). Such medical conditions must be acknowledged and planned for accordingly.

Conclusions

Even though MO is quite prevalent in people with disabilities, orthodontic treatment is still considered an elective procedure. This is owed to the significant challenges in terms of behaviour management, training, expertise and parent/patient cooperation that may be encountered. Orthodontic treatment requires a steadfast commitment on part of both the practitioner and the patient/parent as it involves protracted periods of time, long appointments, dealing with foreign devices in and around the mouth and a diligent attention to oral hygiene. Regular orthodontic treatment paradigms may have to be adapted to suit the unique situation of patients with SHCNs which requires commitment and expertise. It may require undertaking procedures under sedation/general anaesthesia along with a multidisciplinary approach to the patient's oral health issues. When rendered effectively, orthodontic treatment can produce a significant change in the patient's social integration and acceptance as well as improve oral function and overall aesthetics.

References

Baek, S. H., Moon, H. S., & Yang, W. S. (2002). Cleft type and Angle's classification of malocclusion in Korean cleft patients. *The European Journal of Orthodontics, 24*(6), 647–653.

Becker, A., & Shapira, J. (1996). Orthodontics for the handicapped child. *European Journal of Orthodontics, 18*, 55–67.

Becker, A., Chaushu, S., & Shapira, J. (2004). Orthodontic treatment for the special needs child. In *Seminars in orthodontics* (Vol. 10, No. 4, pp. 281–292). WB Saunders.

Becker, A., Shapira, J., & Chaushu, S. (2001). Orthodontic treatment for disabled children–a survey of patient and appliance management. *Journal of Orthodontics, 28*(1), 39–44. https://doi.org/10.1093/ortho/28.1.39.

Becker, A., Shapira, J., & Chaushu, S. (2009). Orthodontic treatment for the special needs child. *Progress in Orthodontics, 10*(1), 34–47.

Brown, J. P., & Schodel, D. R. (1976). A review of controlled surveys of dental disease in handicapped persons. *ASDC Journal of Dentistry for Children, 43*(5), 313–320.

Cabrita, J. P., Bizarra, M. D. F., & Graca, S. R. (2017). Prevalence of malocclusion in individuals with and without intellectual disability: A comparative study. *Special Care in Dentistry, 37*(4), 181–186.

Chaushu, S., Shapira, J., & Becker, A. (2012). Orthodontic treatment for the special needs child. *Integrated Clinical Orthodontics*, 485–499.

Oreland, A., Heijbel, J., & Jagell, S. (1987). Malocclusions in physically and/or mentally handicapped children. *Swedish Dental Journal, 11*(3), 103–119.

Rada, R., Bakhsh, H. H., & Evans, C. (2015). Orthodontic care for the behavior-challenged special needs patient. *Special Care in Dentistry: Official Publication of the American Association of Hospital Dentists, the Academy of Dentistry for the Handicapped, and the American Society for Geriatric Dentistry, 35*(3), 138–142. https://doi.org/10.1111/scd.12082.

Shapira, J., Becker, A., & Moskovitz, M. (1999). The management of drooling problems in children with neurological dysfunction: A review and case report. *Special Care in Dentistry: Official Publication of the American Association of Hospital Dentists, the Academy of Dentistry for the Handicapped, and the American Society for Geriatric Dentistry, 19*(4), 181–185. https://doi.org/10.1111/j.1754-4505.1999.tb01382.x.

Shyama, M., al-Mutawa, S. A., & Honkala, S. (2001). Malocclusions and traumatic injuries in disabled schoolchildren and adolescents in Kuwait. *Special Care in Dentistry: Official Publication of the American Association of Hospital Dentists, the Academy of Dentistry for the Handicapped, and the American Society for Geriatric Dentistry, 21*(3), 104–108. https://doi.org/10.1111/j.1754-4505.2001.tb00235.x.

Utomi, I. L., & Onyeaso, C. O. (2009). Malocclusion and orthodontic treatment need of mentally handicapped children in Lagos, Nigeria.

Vignehsa, H., Soh, G., Lo, G. L., & Chellappah, N. K. (1991). Dental health of disabled children in Singapore. *Australian Dental Journal, 36*(2), 151–156. https://doi.org/10.1111/j.1834-7819.1991.tb01345.x.

Vittek, J., Winik, S., Winik, A., Sioris, C., Tarangelo, A. M., & Chou, M. (1994). Analysis of orthodontic anomalies in mentally retarded developmentally disabled (MRDD) persons. *Special Care in Dentistry : Official Publication of the American Association of Hospital Dentists, the Academy of Dentistry for the Handicapped, and the American Society for Geriatric Dentistry, 14*(5), 198–202. https://doi.org/10.1111/j.1754-4505.1994.tb01131.x.

Winter, K., Baccaglini, L., & Tomar, S. (2008). A review of malocclusion among individuals with mental and physical disabilities. *Special Care in Dentistry: Official Publication of the American Association of Hospital Dentists, the Academy of Dentistry for the Handicapped, and the American Society for Geriatric Dentistry, 28*(1), 19–26. https://doi.org/10.1111/j.1754-4505.2008.00005.x.

Concluding Remarks

Abstract The literature on oral health and disability has picked up in recent years which shows an increased interest in this section of the population. Overall, the general fact is that people with special needs require individualised treatment plans, considerations for accessibility as well as communication. Research in this domain needs to be standardised in its reporting in terms of defining people with disabilities and special needs, amongst other things. Greater advocacy for dental or oral health care in such individuals will hopefully lead to a more rapid and effective integration of these individuals into not only health care but society as a whole as well.

Keywords Disability · Special needs · Research · Advocacy

As is evident from the preceding sections of this text, oral health forms a significant aspect of the lives of people with disabilities. Oral health-related diseases and conditions such as periodontal disease, caries, dental trauma and malocclusion cause a significant burden of disease in people with disabilities. The problem is compounded by issues of accessibility and communication which may pose significant challenges in these patients.

Disabilities present in varying forms and severity which makes the condition of each individual unique. This may further be complicated by social, economic and psychological factors. It is important for practitioners to realise these issues and tailor their practice, approach and treatment plan accordingly. This can further be enhanced by instituting academic programmes in Special Care Dentistry at the graduate as well as postgraduate level to have a workforce which is trained and motivated in dealing with such patients and the many challenges they face.

The establishment of Special Care Dentistry as a separate branch in the UK is a welcome step. However, this is not the case in a number of countries where no training is provided to dental students in dealing with patients with special needs. Introducing course curriculum changes to incorporate such practices can help in aiding the gap in care as well as train future academicians to impart education in this domain.

There are a number of concerns surrounding research into the oral health of people with disabilities. A large set of studies tend to primarily evaluate the prevalence of certain dental conditions in a broadly defined group of 'people with disabilities' or 'people with special needs'. There is simply too much variation in terms of the disabilities considered, the age groups studied, geographical location, living conditions and so on. There needs to be standardised reporting which may only be beneficial if done on a large scale, in a multi-centric manner. There is also a severe shortage of literature which deals with specific approaches of managing patients with special needs surrounding a particular oral disease or condition. A cookbook approach cannot be successful in every patient seeing as how each is unique in their presentation.

There is also a shortage of literature and guidelines surrounding accessibility in people with disabilities seeking dental care. If society has to integrate people with disabilities in the mainstream, it should not cherry-pick. A set of accessibility norms at the national and international levels should be validated and implemented across the board, and efforts should be made to make dental product manufacturers compliant to making products which mandatorily promote accessibility features. In not doing so, perhaps those with disabilities are being excluded from mainstream health care at least.

A positive sign appears to be the increase over time in the research surrounding those with special needs seeking oral health care as is evidenced by more published research. There appears to be an effort in some societies to make the environment and services more accessible. Greater advocacy will help in furthering this cause in countries and regions where these aspects of life take a back seat or are perhaps non-existent.